Marijuana

Recent Titles in the
CONTEMPORARY WORLD ISSUES
Series

CRIMINAL JUSTICE
Modern Piracy: A Reference Handbook
David F. Marley

GENDER AND ETHNICITY
Women and Crime: A Reference Handbook
Judith A. Warner

POLITICS, LAW, AND GOVERNMENT
Tax Reform: A Reference Handbook, Second Edition
James John Jurinski

Military Robots and Drones: A Reference Handbook
Paul J. Springer

SCIENCE, TECHNOLOGY, AND MEDICINE
Medical Tourism: A Reference Handbook
Kathy Stolley and Stephanie Watson

World Energy Crisis: A Reference Handbook
David E. Newton

SOCIETY
The Rising Costs of Higher Education: A Reference Handbook
John R. Thelin

World Sports: A Reference Handbook
Maylon Hanold

Books in the **Contemporary World Issues** series address vital issues in today's society such as genetic engineering, pollution, and biodiversity. Written by professional writers, scholars, and nonacademic experts, these books are authoritative, clearly written, up-to-date, and objective. They provide a good starting point for research by high school and college students, scholars, and general readers as well as by legislators, businesspeople, activists, and others.

Each book, carefully organized and easy to use, contains an overview of the subject, a detailed chronology, biographical sketches, facts and data and/or documents and other primary source material, a forum of authoritative perspective essays, annotated lists of print and nonprint resources, and an index.

Readers of books in the Contemporary World Issues series will find the information they need in order to have a better understanding of the social, political, environmental, and economic issues facing the world today.

Marijuana

A REFERENCE HANDBOOK

David E. Newton

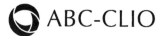 ABC-CLIO

Santa Barbara, California • Denver, Colorado • Oxford, England

Copyright 2013 by ABC-CLIO, LLC

All rights reserved. No part of this publication may be reproduced, stored in a retrieval system, or transmitted, in any form or by any means, electronic, mechanical, photocopying, recording, or otherwise, except for the inclusion of brief quotations in a review, without prior permission in writing from the publisher.

Library of Congress Cataloging-in-Publication Data

Newton, David E.

Marijuana : a reference handbook / David E. Newton.

p. ; cm. — (Contemporary world issues)

Includes bibliographical references and index.

ISBN 978–1–61069–149–9 (alk. paper) — ISBN 978–1–61069–150–5 (ebook)

I. Title. II. Series: Contemporary world issues.

[DNLM: 1. Cannabis. 2. Cannabinoids—therapeutic use. 3. Government Regulation. 4. Marijuana Smoking—legislation & jurisprudence. QV 766]

615.7′827—dc23   2012036276

ISBN: 978–1–61069–149–9

EISBN: 978–1–61069–150–5

17 16 15 14 13   1 2 3 4 5

This book is also available on the World Wide Web as an eBook.

Visit www.abc-clio.com for details.

ABC-CLIO, LLC

130 Cremona Drive, P.O. Box 1911

Santa Barbara, California 93116-1911

This book is printed on acid-free paper ∞

Manufactured in the United States of America

Contents

Preface

Cannabis sativa is one of the oldest crop plants known to humans. One form of the plant known as hemp has been used for the production of textiles, rope, canvas, paper, and other products for at least 6,000 years, and probably much longer. Another form of the plant, known by a variety of names such as *marijuana* and *hashish,* has been a part of religious and mystical ceremonies for just as long. It has an especially long cultural tradition in India, where the Hindu god Siva is said to have sought comfort after a family quarrel by resting under a cannabis plant and eating its leaves. The story explains Siva's alternate name of the Lord of Bhang (bhang being a particular concoction containing marijuana).

Marijuana has also been used for centuries as a recreational drug, a mind-altering substance that allows users to experience a form of the world around them often very different from that experienced in daily life. Archaeological research has found evidence of vessels apparently used for smoking marijuana that date as far back as the first millennium CE in places as widespread as China, India, Assyria, and Africa. The use of marijuana as a recreational drug persists today, with the UN Office on Drugs and Crime reporting in 2011 that there were an estimated 125 to 203 million individuals worldwide who had used the drug for recreational purposes at least once in the previous year.

For most of human history, cannabis has been held in high regard for all of these applications. It has been praised as one of the most durable, attractive, and useful of all fabrics; it has been honored as a gateway to spiritual insights; and it has been cherished as a relaxing release from the troubles of everyday life, which is not to say that questions have not been raised about possible harmful effects of the plant and its derivatives. Indeed, at the very times cannabis was most popular in some cultures as a source of clothing, a sacramental herb, or a healing medication, some individuals and groups have warned about the damage cannabis can cause to the human body and mind. At one time in ancient China, for example, laws were passed prohibiting the use of marijuana for certain purposes because in people who used it the most, it tended to bring out riotous aspects of their personalities, thus posing a possible threat to peace and order in the general society.

Such concerns have often led to conferences, conventions, and other meetings at which experts reassess the possible benefits and risks of using various forms of cannabis (usually, marijuana and hashish). Interestingly enough, these meetings have almost always concluded with a renewed statement of the many benefits provided by the cannabis plant and limited warnings about the risks of overexposure to the drug. Committee reports, like those of the Indian Hemp Drug Commission of 1895, almost always say that cannabis products do no physical, mental, or moral harm; may actually be good for you; and are safe, even "far safer than many foods we commonly consume," according to one official of the U.S. Drug Enforcement Administration (DEA) in 1988.

And yet in the second decade of the 21st century, the use of cannabis and its derivatives is illegal in almost every nation in the world. Beginning in the early 20th century, a movement to change public views about the use of cannabis products began to develop, perhaps most strongly in the United States, but in other parts of the world also. International meetings, such as the International Opium Convention of 1912, were called to develop strategies for limiting or banning the production, transport, and consumption of cannabis products throughout the world. Penalties for the use of such products were severe, sometimes more severe than penalties for other major crimes, such as rape, assault, and armed burglary. Such penalties are still in existence in some parts of the world; drug trafficking can result in the death penalty in some countries, and prison sentences of up to 20 years for possession of cannabis are still place in some states of the United States.

What happened to bring about this dramatic change in official attitudes about hemp, marijuana, and other cannabis products in the early 20th century? How did this revered plant go from being regarded as a blessing to human civilization to one of the most reviled products in the world? That question is one of the themes of this book because it helps to inform the current debate over cannabis in the world today. This debate focuses at its most fundamental level on the question of whether cannabis should be criminalized at all and, if so, under what circumstances. On a somewhat more limited, but equally important and controversial, level the debate has to do with the use of marijuana and related substances for medical purposes.

The purpose of this book is to provide an introduction to the topic of marijuana. Chapter 1 provides a general background about the science of the plant and its history in human civilization. Chapter 2 focuses on the two major disputes over cannabis in today's world: should cannabis products be legally available and, if so, under what conditions, and should a special dispensation be allowed for the use of medical marijuana, regardless of general laws and regulations regarding the personal use of the substance? The remaining chapters of the book provide background information for readers who wish to continue their study of these issues in more detail. Chapter 3 provides some statements pro and con on the legality of marijuana in general and for medical purposes. Chapter 4 offers profiles of some important individuals and organizations that have been involved in the debates over cannabis both in recent years and in earlier history. Chapter 5 is a collection of some especially important documents—laws, policy statements, and court decisions—related to marijuana issues, as well as data on production and consumption of marijuana products. Chapter 6 provides an annotated list of books, articles, and reports, as well as electronic resources on marijuana. Chapter 7 is a timeline of important events in the history of marijuana, and the book ends with a glossary of basic terms used in discussions of cannabis and related products.

Marijuana

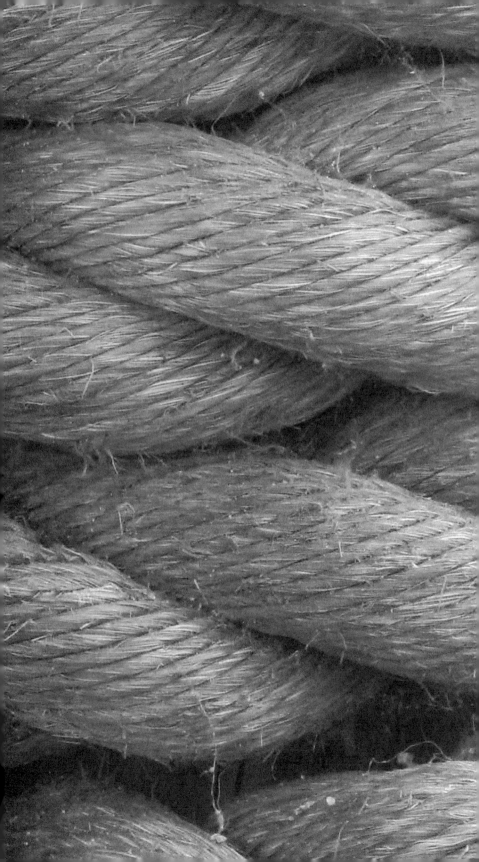

The researchers were not quite sure what to make of their discovery. The pottery shards they had found in their excavations at Yangmingshan, close to modern Taipei, Taiwan, were obviously very old. And the decorations on the pottery had clearly been made by some type of rope. But what was the rope made of? It was certainly one of the oldest woven materials the archaeologists had ever seen. Could it be that the fiber used to decorate the pots was the oldest material of its kind in human history?

As it turned out, this discovery was as exciting as the researchers had hoped it would be. Further analysis proved that the rope used to decorate the pottery fragments was made of hemp, a material made from the plant now known as *Cannabis sativa*. Carbon dating of the fibers found that the hemp was about 12,000 years old, dating back to a Neolithic society known as the Tapenkeng culture (Booth 2005, 20). So, yes, the hemp found in this archaeological dig may well be the oldest fiber ever produced by humans.

What Is *Cannabis Sativa*?

This story from Neolithic Taiwan provides just a hint of the very long history of an amazing plant, *Cannabis sativa*. Before

Hemp has many commercial applications, including the manufacture of building materials, plastic alternatives, fuels, fabrics and textiles, and cordage, as shown in this photograph. (morgueFile.com)

continuing that story, it is necessary to describe in more detail that plant, now commonly known simply as cannabis (sometimes correctly spelled with a capital "C," as Cannabis, but more commonly spelled with a lower case "c," as cannabis).

As its scientific name suggests, *Cannabis sativa* belongs to the genus *Cannabis*, in the family Cannabaceae (also known as the hemp family), the order Urticales, the class Magnoliopsida (the dicotyledons), and the division Magnoliophyta (the flowering plants). The species is named is often written as *Cannabis sativa L.*, with the capital "L" representing the name of the person who originally named the plant, Linnaeus. There is some disagreement among experts as to the number of species in the genus Cannabis, with some authorities recognizing two other species in addition to *C. sativa*: *C. indica* and *C. ruderalis*. Many taxonomists argue that *C. indica* and *C. ruderalis* are subspecies of *C. sativa*, rather than true species themselves. Many taxonomic listings of the genus show both classifications for *C. indica* and *C. ruderalis*. *C. sativa* is thought to have originated in eastern Asia, although some authorities claim that it may also have developed in Africa or parts of the Americas.

C. sativa is an annual flowering dioecious herb with erect stems that may reach a height of five meters (about 16 feet). The term *dioecious* means that the plant may occur as male or female, in contrast to monecious plants, which have both male and female parts on the same plant. The dioecious character of the cannabis plant was recognized as early as the third century BCE by Chinese naturalists, who called the male plant *xi* and the female plant *fu*. (The Chinese name for cannabis itself is *ma*.) Reproduction of the cannabis plant, then, can occur only when male and female plants are in proximity to each other so that microspores from the male plant can be transferred to the megaspores of a second (female) plant. The plant typically flowers in the summer and produces its fruit in late summer to early fall. It grows year-around in the tropics but is a deciduous annual in temperate regions.

Cannabis belongs to a family of plants known as *short-day plants*, plants that require some given amount of darkness in order to flower. Flowering does not occur if nights are not long enough, that is, if there is too much daylight within a 24-hour period. Flowering of a short-day plant can be inhibited, for example, simply by shining a bright light on the plant in the middle of the night, thus interrupting the period of darkness it requires for flowering. This characteristic explains the tendency of cannabis plants to begin flowering later in the summer (after the summer solstice, on or about June 21).

The *C. sativa* plant is often described as "leggy" because it has long branches with large narrow-bladed leaves. The plant also has large internodal distances. The internodal distance on a plant is the space between two nodes on a stem (a node is the point at which an individual leaf grows off the stem). The plant has a large, sprawling root system.

The cannabis fruit is usually a shiny brown achene (a small, dry fruit with a single distinct interior seed) that may be either plain in color or marked in a variety of ways. At maturation, it detaches from the plant and is blown away, the mechanism by which the plant reproduces.

The subspecies *C. indica* differs from *C. sativa* in a number of ways. First, it tends to be shorter and bushier than the main species, with a more compact root system. Its leaves are broader, a darker green, and more densely arranged on the plant than in *C. sativa*. These traits tend to make it more popular among growers who have a limited amount of space in which to locate their plants, such as indoor growers. The subspecies also has distinctly different pharmacological effects than those experienced with the main species (see later in this chapter). *C. indica* is thought to have originated on the Indian subcontinent.

The subspecies *C. ruderalis* is even smaller and more compact than *C. indica*. It is a scrubby plant of little interest to marijuana growers because it has a very low concentration of tetrahydrocannabinol (THC; the primary active ingredient in the Cannabis plant), tending to produce headaches rather than the more pleasant effects obtained by ingesting *C. sativa* or *C. indica*. *C. ruderalis* is thought to have originated in Russia, Central Europe, or Central Asia and was first introduced to the modern world when seeds were brought to Amsterdam in the 1980s.

The three forms of cannabis discussed thus far have been variously called distinct species, species and subspecies, species and strains, or species and varieties. Strains and varieties are forms of a plant that differ from each other in important characteristics, but that do not differ sufficiently to be assigned distinct taxa. For example, cannabis growers typically attempt to produce new strains (or varieties) by pollinating one form of *C. sativa, C. indica*, or *C. ruderalis* with a second form of one of the three varietals. The purpose of such experiments is to produce new types of cannabis that have especially desirable qualities favored by users of the plant. Today, there are well over 100 different strains of the cannabis plant that have been produced by years of this crossbreeding technology (Oner 2011, xi). Some of those strains are called Afghani, Amsterdam Indica, Aussie Blues, Big Bud, Charas, Durban Poison, Haze Marijuana, Island Lady, Kush, Light of Jah, Mauwie Wauwie, New York Diesel, Purple Haze Marijuana, Super Skunk, Swiss Miss, and White Queen. Many strains are developed because they grow best in either indoor or outdoor settings.

Among individuals for whom the cannabis plant is a source of a recreational drug (marijuana), probably the most interesting and important part of the plant is the trichome. A trichome is a small hair or other outgrowth from the epidermis of a plant, usually consisting of a single cell. Trichomes typically exude a sticky, resinous substance to which bits of dust, male sex spores, small insects, and other materials become stuck. Botanists have hypothesized that the primary evolutionary purpose of trichomes is as part of the plants' defensive system, protecting them from attacking insects (Freeman and Beattie 2011). Research indicates that chemicals found in the exudate of trichomes are toxic to insects that prey on the plant.

A number of important organic compounds occur at the base of a trichome, including a number of phenols and terpenes. Phenols are organic compounds related to phenol (hydroxybenzene), a ring compound with one hydroxyl (-OH) group. The chemical formula for phenol is C_6H_5OH. Terpenes are organic compounds that occur very commonly in plants. They constitute a large and diverse collection of compounds derived from the simply unsaturated hydrocarbon isoprene (2-methyl-1,3-butadiene; C_5H_8). As phenols and terpenes migrate upward from the base of a trichome to the bud at its tip, a series of chemical reactions occur that convert these simple basic compounds into a large variety of more complex compounds, the most important of which is Δ-9-tetrahydrocannabinol, also known simply as tetrahydrocannabinol, (Δ^9-THC), or THC. THC is a light yellow resinous oil that is sticky at room temperature and solidifies upon refrigeration. It is virtually insoluble in water but soluble in most organic solvents. THC is of interest both to scientists and to users of marijuana because it is the most psychoactive of the many compounds found in the cannabis plant. It is also of interest to chemists because it is the only known psychoactive plant material that does not contain the element nitrogen. Overall, more than 400 distinct chemicals have been extracted from the cannabis plant, 66 of which are unique to that plant ("Definitions and Explanations" 2011). These 66 chemicals are collectively known as *cannabinoids*. Many cannabinoids are isomers of each other, that is, they have the same chemical formula (such as that of THC: $C_{21}H_{30}O_2$) but different arrangements of atoms. Table 1.1 gives the names and abbreviations of the classes of cannabinoids found in the cannabis plant.

One of the most interesting discoveries made by researchers in the last few decades is that animals produce compounds with properties similar to those of the cannabinoids that occur in plants (the so-called *phytocannabinoids*). These animal-based compounds are called *endocannabinoids*. They appear to operate on almost every part of an animal's body and brain,

Table 1.1   Cannabinoids Present in the Cannabis Plant

Class of Cannabinoid	Abbreviation
Δ^9-tetrahydrocannabinol	Δ^9-THC; THC
Δ^8-tetrahydrocannabinol	Δ^8-THC
cannabichromene	CBC
cannabicyclol	CBL
cannabidiol	CBD
cannabielsoin	CBE
cannabigerol	CBG
cannabinidiol	CBND
cannabinol	CBN
cannabitriol	CBT
cannabichromanone	CBCN
isocannabinoids	—

producing effects similar to those caused by THC and other phytocannabinoids.

Researchers believe that endocannabinoids may have a number of medical and pharmacological applications because they stimulate the same receptors in the nervous system as those affected by phytocannabinoids. For example, the first commercial product to emerge from research on endocannabinoids is a drug called rimonabant (Acomplia), which is used in the treatment of obesity. The drug works by blocking the action of endocannabinoids produced by the brain that stimulate a person's appetite ("Information on Acomplia" 2011).

In addition to the naturally occurring cannabinoids, a number of synthetic cannabinoids have been produced by researchers. These compounds do not necessarily exist naturally in plants, but they have many of the same physiological and pharmacological properties as do naturally occurring cannabinoids. One reason for the preparation of synthetic cannabinoids is to study with more specificity their effects on body systems. The result of this research may be helpful in developing synthetic products that can be used to treat a variety of physical and mental conditions. Probably the best known synthetic cannabinoid is a compound called dronabinol, manufactured by United Pharmaceuticals, Inc. Dronabinol is chemically identical to the active form of THC found in cannabis. It is sold under the trade name of Marinol and is recommended for the treatment of anorexia associated with weight loss in patients with HIV/AIDS and for the nausea and vomiting associated with cancer chemotherapy in patients who have not responded to other treatments ("Marinol" 2011). Dronabinol is listed as a schedule III drug by the U.S. Food and Drug Administration (FDA) because it is regarded as a non-narcotic with low risk of physical or mental dependency. That listing has drawn some attention and comment since the synthetic compound dronabinol is chemically identical to the form of THC that is regarded as the most psychoactive component of natural marijuana ("Cannabis/Marijuana" 2011).

A second synthetic cannabinoid is nabilone, marketed as Cesamet and listed by the FDA as a schedule II drug because of its high potential for abuse. Like dronabinol, nabilone is used almost exclusively for treating the nausea and vomiting associated with cancer chemotherapy ("Cesamet" 2011).

Another interesting analog of THC that research chemists developed has the chemical name 1-pentyl-3-(1-naphthoyl) indole, although it is more commonly known as AM-678 or JWH-018 or, commercially, as K2 or Spice. The compound was first synthesized by John W. Huffman, an organic chemist at Clemson University. It has essentially the same effect (except more powerful) on cannabinoid receptors in the body as does THC, although its chemical structure is significantly different. An herbal incense ("not for human consumption") called Spice that contains JWH-018 first appeared in Europe in 2004 and rapidly became popular there. When authorities analyzed the product and found that it contained a powerful synthetic cannabinoid, they banned it. The FDA has since classified JWH-018 as a schedule I substance, making its use in the United States illegal (Stafford 2011).

Hemp versus Marijuana

In today's world, two forms of cannabis are grown for quite different purposes. Both forms are classified botanically as *C. sativa*, but their physical appearances and other properties are different from each other. The form known as *hemp* is usually tall, ranging in height from one to more than five meters (three to nearly 20 feet). Plant appearance depends on the conditions under which it is grown. In uncrowded conditions, a plant has many branches and a relatively thick stalk that can reach more than 50 millimeters (two inches) in diameter. In crowded conditions, the hemp plant has few branches, except at the very top. The stalk is much reduced in size, with a diameter of no more than about 20 millimeters (about 0.75 inch).

Hemp is grown for two purposes: fibers, which are made from the plant's stalk and stems, and oil, which is made from its seeds. The manufacture of fiber from the hemp plant begins with a process known as *retting*, in which stalks and stems are soaked in water that contains bacteria or special kinds of chemicals. These bacteria or chemicals attack the stems and stalks, breaking them down into their component parts. One of those parts is called *bast* or *bast fiber*, a material found between the woody core of the plant and its outer covering (the epidermis and cortex). Bast fibers are long stringy strands up to two meters (six feet) in length that provide the hemp plant with strength and that, when separated from the rest of the plant, produce strong, durable fibers. These fibers tend to be yellowish, pale green, or gray in color and are not easily dyed, accounting for the pale color associated with most hemp fibers. The fibers are used for a host of purposes, including the manufacture of all styles of clothing, paper, ropes and other types of cordage, sail canvas, and netting. Hemp has long been a popular agricultural crop because it grows quickly, requires little fertilizer or pesticide application, produces large yields per acre compared to other plants, and has few deleterious environmental impacts.

A second use of the hemp plant is the production of oil, which is made from the plant's seeds. Growing hemp for oil production cannot be combined with growing hemp for fiber production because in the latter process, plants are harvested before they begin to flower; thus no seeds are produced that can be used for oil production. Hemp plants destined for use in oil production must be allowed to grow a few weeks longer than those used for fiber production, permitting the growth of flowers and the development of seeds. When this point has been reached, the seeds are harvested and then pressed to produce an oil that is similar to safflower, linseed, tung, and perilla oils. Freshly prepared unrefined hempseed oil is light green to dark green in color with a pleasant nutty aroma. It is rich in unsaturated fatty acids and has significant nutritional value. But it is also a fragile material that must be stored in dark, cool, oxygen-free conditions to prevent breakdown. Because of its instability, hempseed oil also cannot be used for cooking. Its nutritional value, however, has made it popular, especially among natural and organic food devotees, as a nutritional supplement that can be used as a condiment and in the preparation of sauces and specialized foods such as pesto.

In some ways, the most important feature of the hemp plant is its concentration of THC. Over the centuries, the hemp plant has been crossbred to have low concentrations of THC, presently about 0.3 percent. By contrast, cannabis plants raised for the production of marijuana have much higher concentrations of THC, ranging from about 2 to as much as 20 percent. Somewhat ironically, this dramatic difference in THC content in hemp and marijuana plants is irrelevant to federal laws in the United States, where plants containing any amount of THC greater than zero are illegal ("DEA Clarifies Status of Hemp" 2011). Thus neither hemp nor marijuana plants may legally be grown in the United States (except with special permits granted for specific purposes). Laws in some states of the United States and in other countries differ on this point. A half dozen U.S. states have passed laws permitting the growing of hemp, but those laws have not yet gone into force because of their conflict with federal law, and the growing of hemp is legal in any foreign country.

One form of hemp that is still found in the United States is called *feral hemp* or *ditchweed* (or *ditch weed*). Feral hemp, as the name suggests, is hemp that has self-seeded from plants that were once grown legally in virtually every part of the United States at one time. They are vigorous plants that have survived many decades of attempted eradication. Interestingly enough, up to 99 percent of all marijuana plants eradicated annually by the U.S. Drug Enforcement Administration (DEA) are not those cultivated intentionally for the production of marijuana; rather, they are feral plants ("98 Percent Of All Domestically Eradicated Marijuana" 2011). In 2005, for example, the DEA eradicated a total of 218,633,492 feral plants (with no THC value) compared to 4,209,086 plants they eradicated that were being grown intentionally for harvesting of marijuana ("Sourcebook of Criminal Justice Statistics" 2011).

The Cannabis Plant in Early China

Whatever the diverse forms in which it is currently found, *C. sativa* almost certainly existed as only a single type of plant when it was first used by humans. The date of that first use, as noted previously, was at least 10,000 BCE on the modern island of Taiwan. Much of what we know about the early history of cannabis comes from China, where the plant became widely popular with the rise of Chinese civilization. Indeed, in some of the oldest documents available, ancient China was sometimes referred to as the Land of Mulberry and Hemp (Booth 2005, 20). An archaeological find of some interest that is similar to the Taiwanese discovery was reported in 1974. It consisted of a number of artifacts indicating the use of hemp in the culture of the time, including a design on pottery similar to that found in Taiwan and some imprints made from hemp clothing on the then-damp pottery (Merlin 2003, 304).

Like the Taiwan discovery, the earliest evidence for the use of hemp in China comes from archaeological digs in which remnants of cloth, seeds, rope imprints (like those from the Taiwan site), and other visual evidence of the plant and its use are available. For example, a fragment of cloth made from hemp was discovered in 1972 in a grave dating to the Zhou dynasty (1045–256 BCE). The find is sometimes described as the "oldest preserved specimen" of hemp cloth ever discovered (Hanuš and Mechoulam 2008, 50). Many other hemp products have also been recovered from ancient Chinese sites. Fragments of textiles made from hemp have been discovered at a site at Anyang in Henan Province dating to the Shan dynasty (1600–1046 BCE), and cemeteries at the same site dating to the Zhou dynasty contain thousands of funerary objects, some of which are made of hemp. Excavations in Gansu Province have discovered graves dating to the Han dynasty (206 BCE–220 CE) in which corpses were wrapped in cloth made of hemp (Fleming and Clarke 1998, 87).

Written records of the role of hemp in Chinese culture began to appear as early as the 16th century BCE when it was listed as an important crop in what is regarded as the oldest Chinese agricultural manuscript, the *Xia Xiao Zheng*. The role of hemp in agriculture was also mentioned and described in other early documents. These documents include the *Shi Ching* (*Book of Songs*) and the *Zhushu Jinian* (*Bamboo Annals*), both written between 476 and 221 BCE; *Shi Jing* (*Book of Odes*), dating to the eleventh to sixth centuries BCE; *Si Min Yue Ling* (Eastern Han dynasty; 25–220 CE); and *Qi Min Yao Shu* (Northern Wei dynasty; 386–534 CE). All of these texts provided detailed information about the planting and cultivation of hemp plants, indicating their essential role in Chinese culture (Fleming and Clarke 1998, 87). An example of the kind of instruction found in these books is the following.

If we pull out the male hemp before it scatters pollen, the female plant cannot make seed. Otherwise, the female plant's seed production will be influenced by the male hemp plants scattering pollen and during this period of time, the fiber of the male hemp plant is the best. (Cited in Lu and Clarke, 1995. This article contains a number of other passages dealing with the cultivation of cannabis for the production of hemp.)

A considerable body of evidence indicates that hemp seed was also used as an essential part of the diet among the early Chinese. Early histories and other documents list hemp seed as one of the essential nine (in some references) or five (in other references) grains that constituted a typical diet. Although it was certainly part of the average Chinese diet for many centuries, it also seems to have been a specialty food among the royalty during certain months of the year (Li 1974a, 443). The seed was also crushed to obtain its oil, which was used both for frying foods and industrial applications. Over time, the use of hemp seed as a food and a source of oil was gradually phased out as superior natural products became available. An interesting side note, however, is that a resurgence of the use of hemp seed occurred at one point in history, around 28 CE, when a great famine caused by war and natural disasters forced people to return to the ancient practice of eating hemp seeds as a major part of their diets (Li 1974a, 444). As late as the ninth century CE, writers were still describing a porridge made with cannabis seeds, but before long, the product "was completely forgotten as a human food" (Li 1974a, 444).

Given the widespread use of cannabis as a food, it is hardly surprising that humans would rather quickly recognize the plant's medical and psychoactive effects. One could hardly consume cannabis seeds without experiencing at least some kinds of mind-altering events from time to time. The first mention of cannabis as a medical product is usually given as about 2000 BCE, when it is described in the earliest known pharmacopeia, the *Pe'n-ts'ao Ching*, attributed to the legendary emperor Shen Nung. That attribution is almost certainly wrong since

Shen Nung was probably not a real person, and the oldest known copy of the book actually dates to the first or second century CE. However, authorities believe that the text accurately reflects prehistoric practices, as its "earliest" mention of medical cannabis is usually taken as valid.

In any case, Chinese shaman used virtually every part of the cannabis plant to treat a variety of illnesses. A 1911 text on Chinese herbal medicine, for example, notes that "[e]very part of the hemp plant is used in medicine; the dried flowers, the ach'enia, the seeds, the oil, the leaves, the stalk, the root, and the juice" (Smith 1911). These materials were put to a plethora of applications used to treat a long list of illness and disorders, including nausea, vomiting, malaria, beriberi, constipation, rheumatic pains, absent-mindedness, nervous disorders, female disorders (including postpartum depression), ulcers and other eruptions of the skin, scorpion stings, wounds, hair loss, sulfur poisoning, dryness of the throat, and worm infestations (an incomplete list at that!). Concoctions of the plant were also recommended to prevent one from aging and having one's hair turn gray (Smith 1911).

The cannabis plant was also used as an anesthetic for surgical procedures, perhaps as early as the second century CE. Although there is considerable dispute about the details of this history, it appears that the famous Chinese physician Hua Tuo used powdered cannabis in a concoction to produce numbness during surgery. Reputedly, the product used by Hua was made of a concoction of cannabis mixed with wine. It was called *mafeisan*, which means *cannabis* ("ma") *boil* ("fei") *powder* ("san") (The First Anaesthetic in the World 2011; Li 1974a, 446).

The use of the cannabis plant for both medical and psychoactive purposes in ancient history is hardly surprising. A practitioner who purported to heal individuals of physical and mental disorders was commonly a shaman, a person who used minerals, herbs, and other natural products to treat the patient, but who was also in contact with the spirit world and could thus draw on supernatural resources to bring about cures. It has seemed clear to such practitioners perhaps since the beginning of human civilization that the cannabis plant produced both kinds of results: as an herb, it could directly cure a host of physical and mental ailments; as a psychoactive material, it could give a patient or the practitioner access to a world of spirits who could perhaps provide cures on an entirely different psychical plane.

References to the use of cannabis as both a medical substance and a psychoactive material date to the earliest of the Chinese pharmacopoeias, *Pen Ching*. There one can find the following admonition:

> To take too much makes people see demons and throw themselves about like maniacs. But if one takes it over a long period of time one can communicate with the spirits and one's own body becomes light. (as cited in Rudgley 2011)

The fact that the Chinese knew about the hallucinatory effects of cannabis early in history comes, interestingly enough, from linguistic studies. In a 1974 article in *Economic Botany*, Hui-Lin Li of the Morris Arboretum at the University of Pennsylvania points out that the Chinese character for "ma" (the Chinese name for cannabis) is a combination of simpler characters that represent "numerous" or "chaotic," apparently from the nature of hemp fibers themselves, and "numbness" or "senselessness," apparently from the plant's physical effects. He concludes that these linguistic clues indicate "that the stupefying effect of the hemp plant was commonly known from extremely early times" (Li 1974b, 296).

In spite of a number of mentions such as these in early Chinese documents, use of cannabis for psychoactive purposes was probably relatively limited. Observers note that Chinese society was highly ordered, and activities that would disrupt that order were frowned upon and often restricted. As Martin Booth (2005) has written in his history of cannabis:

> The use of cannabis [for recreational purposes], however, never really became more than a passing phase. Chinese culture, being based on social order, family values and the reverence of ancestors and the elderly, looked down upon drugs. (23)

Cannabis in India and Central Asia

The same cannot be said for other parts of Asia. In fact, the use of cannabis products for psychoactive experiences has a long history, dating back to at least 1400 BCE. Historians are uncertain as to the mechanism by which knowledge of the cannabis plant worked its way from China (or, perhaps, Central Asia), but there is no question of the central role that the plant had in Indian culture from its earliest days. The sacred Hindu texts, known as the Vedas, contain many references to the psychoactive effects of the cannabis plant, an effect that is universally praised and encouraged. In one segment of the *Artharvaveda*, for example, cannabis is referred to as one of the herbs that "release us from anxiety" (as cited in Rudgley 2011).

According to one of the central stories told in the Vedas, the cannabis plant first appeared on Earth when a drop of heavenly nectar fell to Earth, took root, and grew as a cannabis plant. A drink prepared from the plant later became the favorite refreshment of Indra, the Hindu Lord of Kings. Another popular myth recounts the experience of Lord Shiva who, after an angry fight within his family, wandered off into the fields and fell asleep under the leaves of a cannabis plant. When he awoke, he decided to slake his hunger by eating a leaf off the plant, and found it to be delicious and refreshing. In later life, he came to be known as the Lord of Bhang because of his love of the plant (Gumbiner 2011).

Bhang is one of a number of forms in which cannabis was (and is) consumed in India. It is a mixture with a variable composition. One that has been described consists of cannabis, poppy seed, pepper, ginger, caraway seed, clove, cardamom, cinnamon, cucumber seed, almonds, nutmeg, and rosebud, all boiled together in milk (Abel 1982, Chapter 1). In this recipe, the cannabis is taken from the large green leaves and flowering shoots of either the male or female plant. Two other cannabis preparations that have been popular throughout history are ganja and charas. Ganja is made from the top leaves and the unfertilized flower of the young female plant, which are then dried and smoked or brewed as a tea. This preparation produces an effect similar to smoking a mild grade of marijuana that is available today. Charas is made from the resin obtained from the top leaves and unfertilized flower of the female plant, which are then dried and smoked. This is the strongest preparation of cannabis available and is comparable in its effects to hashish. Hashish preparations can have some of the highest concentrations of THC of any form of cannabis and have been popular in many parts of the world throughout much of human history ("Hashish" 2011).

Cannabis preparations have traditionally played a role in Indian culture similar to that played by alcohol in Western culture. They are commonly smoked by groups of people who are gathered for social occasions. For example, legend has it that evil spirits hover around wedding ceremonies waiting for an opportunity to cause misery in the lives of the bride and groom. A gift of bhang from the bride's father is considered sufficient protection against these terrible events. Bhang was (and still is) offered to visitors to one's home, and anyone who ignores this tradition is usually regarded as "miserly and misanthropic" (Abel 1982).

Many scholars today believe that cannabis was first domesticated and used not in China or India, but in Central Asia. Martin Booth, author of *Cannabis: A History* (2005), argues that the plant's original home may have been near the Irtysh

River, which flows from Mongolia, along the southern edge of the Gobi Desert, into the lowlands of western Siberia or in the Takla Makan Desert north of Tibet. The plant still grows in abundance in these regions whenever the earth is disturbed by floods or erosion (Booth 2005, 3). In such a case, the plant was probably then dispersed eastward into China and southward into India. One of the most solid pieces of evidence arguing for a long (if not the longest) history of cannabis in Central Asia comes from the writings of the Greek historian Herodotus, who lived from about 484 to about 425 BCE. In his work, *Histories*, Herodotus tells of a popular tradition among the Scythians in which cannabis was smoked for religious, ceremonial, and perhaps recreational purposes. The Scythians thrived from about 600 BCE to about 300 CE across an extensive region that covered most of the southern part of modern Russia. For their ceremonies, the Scythians first built a tent with three long wooden poles tied together at the top and covered with animal skin. They then placed dried cannabis seeds into a hot bowl in the center of the tent and took their places inside the tent around the bowl. In this position, they inhaled the vapors of the roasting cannabis seeds, experiencing such pleasure that, according to Herodotus, "they would howl with pleasure" (cited in Merlin 2003, 313).

Fortunately, it is not necessary to rely just on the words of Herodotus about this custom. In 1929, the Russian archaeologist S. I. Rudenko visited the region in which the Scythians once lived and found that the tradition reported by Herodotus continues today. He reported that these modern descendants of the Scythians follow the traditional practice not for religious or ceremonial reasons, but simply as a form of day-to-day relaxation. Even more recent information about this practice became available in 1993 when a group of Russian archaeologists discovered the body of a 2,000-year-old woman buried in the permafrost in Siberia near the location of Rudenko's research. The archaeologists found the woman buried in a tree trunk along with a small cask containing cannabis seeds, which they hypothesized were "smoked for pleasure and used in pagan rituals" (Spicer 2011; Stanley 1994). A few authorities have argued for a very early appearance of cannabis in the Middle East. In a 1938 book on cannabis— *Marijuana, America's New Drug Problem*—for example, physician and reputed "authority on marijuana" Robert P. Walton referred to mentions on Assyrian tablets of cannabis dating to about 650 BCE, and possibly much earlier (as cited in Brecher 1972, 397). Since this early comment, there have been only a few significant discoveries pointing to an early history of cannabis in the Middle East. In the early 1960s, for example, archaeologists discovered pieces of hemp fabric in a grave mound at a dig in the region known as Gordion that dates to the eighth century BCE. An even more recent and more fascinating discovery was made in the 1990s in the town of Beit Shemesh, near Jerusalem. The discovery consisted of the skeleton of a young woman who was about 14 years of age and had apparently died during childbirth. Interred with the body was a brown material in the abdominal region of the skeleton, whose composition was found to consist of cannabis seeds mixed with fruits and other dried seeds. Archaeologists believe that the mixture was used as an aid in childbirth, a custom that prevailed in the area well into the 19th century. The find raises questions as to the extent and the purposes for which cannabis might have been used in this early Middle Eastern culture. In spite of these recent finds, most authorities seem to believe that cannabis came to the Middle East relatively later than it did to Central Asia, China, and India.

More intriguing, perhaps, has been the dispute as to whether cannabis products are mentioned in the Bible, which would, of course, place their use many centuries and even millennia earlier. The basic problem is whether words used in the Old Testament actually refer to cannabis or to some other type of plant. In I Samuel 14, for example, Saul places a restriction on his people, telling them that they should not eat until he took vengeance upon his enemies. His son Jonathan did not hear that command, however, and when the army reached a wooded area, he

> ... reached out the end of the staff that was in his hand and dipped it into the honeycomb. He raised his hand to his mouth, and his eyes brightened. (I Samuel 14:27)

The question is whether there is more than meets the eye to this seemingly innocuous passage. According to one historian, there may in fact be. In a 1903 article on the passage, Dr. C. Creighton points out that the Hebrew words for "honey comb" used here—*yagarah hadebash*—probably should be translated as a type of flower stalk similar to that of cannabis, and that the "brightened eyes" may have been Jonathan's response to ingesting cannabis (Creighton 1903, 241; for an extended discussion of this point, also see Benet 1975). Other scholars take a more skeptical view of efforts to place the cannabis plant into Biblical sources. One widely respected authority, for example, has criticized experts who have "tickled, teased, and twisted [Biblical texts] into surrendering secret references to marijuana that it never contained" (Abel 1982).

Africa

The use of any form of cannabis on the African continent appears to have been a comparatively recent event. According to the best information now available, cannabis was probably introduced to the continent by Muslim sea traders who brought the plant to the eastern coast of Africa in the first century CE, after which it spread inland throughout most of southern Africa. There are a few scattered reports of ancient remnants of cannabis finds such as a discovery of prehistoric pollen samples dating to about 2300 BCE from the Kalahari Desert in Botswana, but these are rare, with most discoveries dating to only the first century CE or much later (Merlin 2003, 315–316). More commonly, the archeological record appears to confirm that tribesmen practiced a communal use of cannabis by, for example, "throwing hemp plants on the burning coals of a fire and staging what might today be called a 'breathe-in'" (Emboden 1972, 226, as cited in Spicer 2011).

A somewhat minor, but very interesting, note about the use of cannabis products in Africa has to do with a modern organization known as the Ethiopian Zion Coptic Church (EZCC). Modern leaders of the church say that it has been in existence for a long time, with roots in Africa going back hundreds of years. Whatever its ancient history, the church was formulated in its modern form in the 1930s during the rise of the Rastafari movement in Jamaica. Rastafari (also known as Rasta, but not as Rastafarianism) is a religious movement that consists almost entirely of Christian descendants of slaves brought to the Western Hemisphere. They originally worshiped Haile Selassie I, Emperor of Ethiopia from 1930 to 1974, as the reincarnation of Christ and God incarnate. Among the tenets of the church is a belief in the sacramental role of cannabis smoking as a way of communicating with God. One of the early leaders of the church, Louv Williams, said that the church was based on a new trinity consisting of "The Man, The Herb, and The Word" ("the herb" being cannabis) (Menelik 2009, 138). A defense for the fundamental principles of Rastafari and its basis in Biblical teachings was laid out in a 1988 publication, *Marijuana and the Bible*, which contains dozens of specific citations in the Bible that purportedly allude to the use of cannabis in religious ceremonies. The church's fundamental teaching is that

> Herb (marijuana) is a Godly creation from the beginning of the world. It is known as the weed of wisdom, angel's food, the tree of life and even the "Wicked Old Ganja Tree." Its purpose in creation is as a fiery sacrifice to be offered to our Redeemer during obligations. (Ethiopian Zion Coptic Church 1988)

In 1975, a branch of the EZCC consisting primarily of white Americans was incorporated in the state of Florida. Four years later, members of that group were arrested while unloading a large shipment of marijuana from Jamaica, a shipment they said they intended to use in religious ceremonies. The question as to whether the use of marijuana was legal among the members of this religious denomination worked its way through the federal courts over a number of years. Members of the Rafastari argued that their right to use marijuana in their religious ceremonies was protected by the U.S. Constitution's "freedom of religion" clause, which prevents the government from interfering with the religious practices of individuals and denominations. (American Indians are permitted to use the mind-altering drug peyote under this provision of the law.) The U.S. and state governments responded to this argument by saying that the constitutional right to freedom of religion is not absolute but is subject to overweening "public interest" factors such as the risk of a particular drug. In the end, the government's argument won out in the highest court decisions on the Rafastari complaints, and the denomination's right to use marijuana in its ceremonies is not permitted (see, for example, 738 F.2d 497).

One interesting sidelight of this story emerged when an eminent psychiatrist, Brian L. Weiss, chief of the Division of Psychiatry at Mount Sinai Medical Center in New York City, was asked to evaluate 14 members of the EZCC each in Miami and in Jamaica to determine their psychological, physical, and emotional states. Dr. Weiss reported that he was "surprised by the absence of positive findings" among members of both groups. In fact, the only positive finding he could report was that "the American Coptics are functioning at a much better level than they were prior to joining the Coptic Church." He noted that although the number of individuals examined was small, he felt he could conclude that "some people, at least, can smoke marijuana in high doses for sixteen hours daily for up to fifty years without apparent psychological or physical harm" (Weiss 1980).

Cannabis in Europe

As with other parts of the world, cannabis use appears to have a long history in Europe. Perhaps the earliest reference to such use dates to the third millennium BCE in a gravesite near modern-day Bucharest. The gravesite contained small vessels called *pipe cups* that contained burned cannabis seed. Similar finds have been recovered in other parts of Eurasia, prompting the noted Oxford archaeologist Andrew Sherratt to observe that the practice of burning cannabis as a narcotic is a tradition that goes back in this area some 5,000 or 6,000 years and was the focus of social and religious rituals of the pastoral peoples of central Eurasia in prehistoric and early historic times (Goodman, Lovejoy, and Sherratt 2007, 27).

One of the routes by which cannabis may have come to Europe was through the dispersion of the Scythians from their original home in Central Asia into Eastern Europe. Polish anthropologist Sula Benet (also known as Sara Benetowa) has studied this process in some detail. She has noted that the Scythians carried with them the use of cannabis for funerary ceremonies (similar to those described by Herodotus) out of their Central Asian homelands into southern Russia and Eastern Europe over centuries of migration. Some of those customs have been retained into modern times. One such example is the preparation of a soup made of cannabis seeds called *semieniatka* at Christmastime in Poland, Lithuania, and Russia as nourishment for dead souls who have come back to their families at the holidays (Benet 1975).

In his superb review of the history of cannabis, "Archaeological Evidence for the Tradition of Psychoactive Plant Use in the Old World," M. D. Merlin (2003) mentions a number of situations at which various forms of cannabis have been discovered in prehistoric Europe: the Hallstatt and Laténe cultures of Hungary; a site at Vallensbæk in Denmark; in a region near Trier, Germany; and a location at Mikulčice in the Czech Republic, all dating to the Bronze or Iron Ages in Europe (314).

The point at which cannabis reached Western Europe is not known with any certainty. The date most often mentioned for this event is about 500 BCE. An urn containing burnt cannabis seeds found near modern-day Berlin has been carbon-dated to about that period. In any case, a number of references suggest that the plant rapidly dispersed throughout the continent following that date and by the turn of the millennium was used in locations as far west as the British Isles. An instructive story that is often told is that Hieron II, the ruler of Syracuse from 270 to 215 BCE decided to purchase the hemp he needed for his fleet's sails from producers in the Rhone Valley of Germany, rather than the much closer Caspian Sea providers because the former were more skilled and could produce the best hemp available. This story suggests that German growers and producers of hemp must, even as early as the second century BCE, have become highly skilled at working with the plant.

Cannabis probably reached the British Isles in the first century CE. Rope fragments made of hemp have been discovered as far north on the islands as Bar Hill, located between Glasgow and Edinburgh at a fort built by the Romans around 80 CE. By the fourth century, hemp was being grown throughout the British Isles (in contrast to its having been imported by the Romans earlier). At about the same time, the plant was being grown in Scandinavia, where it was being used by the Vikings for the production of sails and ropes. Also within the same period, hemp was apparently being grown and processed in France. This assumption is based on a famous discovery made in the early 1960s with the opening of tombs at the Cathedral of St. Denis in Paris. One of those tombs contained the body of Queen Arnegunde, second wife of King Clothar I, who died in 561. The queen's richly decorated body was wrapped in a cloth made of hemp (Booth 2005, 34–35).

Cannabis arrived in Western Europe by a second route. After the conquest of the Iberian Peninsula by the Moors in 711, the art of papermaking using hemp was brought to Europe from China by way of the new Muslim civilization. By 1150, the first paper mill in Western Europe that was using this technology was constructed in the town of Xatvia in the province of Valencia. Before long, it was exporting paper "to the East and West" (Balfour 1873, 381). Cotton-based paper was being developed at about the same time, but it was found to be generally inferior to hemp-based paper that, by the end of the century, had essentially replaced all cotton-based products. A 19th-century historian reported that some of those earliest hemp-based papers "possess their original qualities even to this day" (Balfour 1873, 381).

By the 16th century, hemp had reached its zenith in Europe, finding use in a host of applications. In the form of paper, it was the material on which such important documents as the *Magna Carta* and Gutenberg's first Bible were printed; in the form of canvas, it was the substance on which most great (and not-so-great) paintings were made; it was the basic material on which shipbuilding depended for sails and ropes of every description; and in many countries, it had become the fabric of choice from which the clothing of commoners was made. A notable observation about the importance of hemp to the 16th-century world can be found in a 1562 book by William Bullein, a relative of King Henry VIII's second wife, Anne Boleyn. Bullein wrote that "no Shippe can sayle without Hempe. . . . No Plowe, or Carte, can be without ropes halters, trace, &c. The Fisher and Fouler must haue Hempe, to make their nettes. And no Archer can wante his bowe string: and the Malt man for his sackes. With it the belle is rong, to seruice in the Church, with many mo thynges profitable" (as quoted in Shrank 2011).

The plant received some small measure of historical fame in the well-known book by the French writer François Rabelais, *Gargantua and Pantagruel,* which devotes three whole chapters to the plant. Rabelais begins by presenting an extended and complete botanical description of the cannabis plant and then provides a paean to its uses:

> Without this herb kitchens would be detested, the tables of dining-rooms abhorred, although there were great plenty

and variety of most dainty and sumptuous dishes of meat set down upon them, and the choicest beds also, how richly soever adorned with gold, silver, amber, ivory, porphyry, and the mixture of most precious metals, would without it yield no delight or pleasure to the reposers in them. . . . In what case would tabellions, notaries, copists, makers of counterpanes, writers, clerks, secretaries, scriveners, and such-like persons be without it? Were it not for it, what would become of the toll-rates and rent-rolls? Would not the noble art of printing perish without it? Whereof could the chassis or paper-windows be made? . . . The altars of Isis are adorned therewith, the Pastophorian priests are therewith clad and accoutred, and whole human nature covered and wrapped therein at its first position and production in and into this world. All the lanific trees of Seres, the bumbast and cotton bushes in the territories near the Persian Sea and Gulf of Bengala, the Arabian swans, together with the plants of Malta, do not all the them clothe, attire, and apparel so many persons as this one herb alone. Soldiers are nowadays much better sheltered under it than they were in former times, when they lay in tents covered with skins. It overshadows the theatres and amphitheatres from the heat of a scorching sun. It begirdeth and encompasseth forests, chases, parks, copses, and groves, for the pleasure of hunters. It descendeth into the salt and fresh of both sea and river-waters for the profit of fishers. By it are boots of all sizes, buskins, gamashes, brodkins, gambadoes, shoes, pumps, slippers, and every cobbled ware wrought and made steadable for the use of man. By it the butt and rover-bows are strung, the crossbows bended, and the slings made fixed. And, as if it were an herb every whit as holy as the vervain, and reverenced by ghosts, spirits, hobgoblins, fiends, and phantoms, the bodies of deceased men are never buried without it. (Rabelais 1894)

In some regards, the most important application of hemp in Western Europe was in the shipbuilding industry. Except for the wood needed for the ship bodies themselves, arguably the most important raw material for ships was hemp, from which sails and ropes were made. Reflecting this importance was a law enacted by King Henry VIII in 1535. In order to provide an adequate supply of hemp for his fleet, Henry required that every landowner sow at least a quarter acre of land to hemp or be fined for the failure to do so (see, as an example, History of Hemp Fibre, 2012). Henry's daughter, Queen Elizabeth, renewed her father's decree in 1563, requiring that any landowner with more than 60 acres plant hemp (Deitch 2003, 12). The practice also spread to Spain, where King Philip announced a similar degree for the nation's widespread lands in both the Old and New Worlds (González 2011; this is a widely cited statement for which a primary source does not appear to be readily available).

The cannabis plant arrived in Western Europe in a very different form—hashish—at a much later date. Hashish is a thick, sticky, dark-colored, sap-like resin made from the flower of the female cannabis plan. It contains the highest concentration of THC of any cannabis product, 20 percent or more (compared to about 5 percent for the average mild marijuana preparation). As with other aspects of the cannabis plant, little is known with certainty about the origins of hashish, although there is little doubt that it was first used in parts of the Middle East (Arabia), perhaps as early as the first century CE. The use of hashish by Qutb ad-Din Haydar, an early saint of the Sufi religion, is one of the best known, if not necessarily entirely accurate, tales of the introduction of hashish to human society ("Hashish History" 2011). According to that story, Haydar, an ascetic monk who never left his home in the mountains, traveled one day into the nearby fields and came across the cannabis plant. When he returned to his home sometime later, his disciples hardly recognized him because of the "air of happiness and whimsey in his demeanor," which was totally inconsistent with his normal personality. He later explained that this change was a result of his having imbibed from the leaves of the cannabis plant, a discovery he ordered the disciples to keep within Sufism ("Hashish History" 2011).

In any case, the use of hashish soon spread throughout the Arab world, where it eventually became, as one writer has said, an "escape hatch for a large segment of Arab society," for whom alcohol was forbidden (Abel 1982; "Hashish and the Arabs" 2012). The drug did not reach Europe, however, until the beginning of the 19th century. Some authorities suggest that the return of French soldiers from Napoleon's army in Egypt at the end of the 18th century was an important mechanism by which the substance was introduced into Europe. In any case, the hashish form of cannabis has never had quite the popularity of the weaker forms of the drug found in marijuana cigarettes. Historically, the most famous hashish-smoking episode has to do with a club of Parisian aristocrats and writers called Le Club des Hachichins (the Hashish Eater's Club), who met on a regular basis at the Hotel de Lauzun for regular hashish smoking event. A number of famous men, including Jacques-Joseph Moreau, Theophile Gautier, Charles Baudelaire, Gérard de Nerval, Eugene Delacroix, and Alexandre Dumas were members of the group. Baudelaire apparently used his experiences at the club as the basis for his later book, *Les Paradis artificiels* (*Artificial Paradises*; 1860), in which he described what it was like to be under the influence of opium and hashish, and argued for drug-taking as a way for humans to understand what a perfect world would be like ("The Hashish Club" 2011).

Cannabis in North America

Most historians doubt that cannabis was native to the Western Hemisphere (probably a correct assumption) or to North America (almost certainly a correct assumption). They tend to believe that the plant arrived in North America by a variety of routes, one of which may have been across the Bering Strait from Siberia. At a time when a land bridge was available across the strait, wandering birds and animals could certainly have carried cannabis seeds with them to the New World (Booth 2005, 38). Some experts suggest that cannabis seeds or hemp products could also have been brought to North America by the Vikings or Chinese explorers dating as far back as the first millennium. The transfer of cannabis from the southern part of the continent (Mexico in particular) is also thought to have been a major route by which the plant entered the region that is now the United States. One of the first goals of the Spanish conquest of South America was to establish new plantations that would provide the vast amounts of hemp that could not be grown in their native country. Those efforts failed in large part because the climate was not suitable for hemp growing, and Spanish masters soon found that the narcotic effects of the plant provided natives with a reasonable excuse for performing poorly in growing and harvesting the crop (Booth 2005, 38).

A century later, a similar scenario was playing out in the new British colonies along the Atlantic coast of North America. Farmers in the mother country, by the early 17th century, could no longer supply even a fraction of the hemp Great Britain needed for its many industrial projects, especially the maintenance of a huge seagoing fleet. The solution seemed to be obvious: establish extensive hemp plantations in the American colonies. As a consequence, most colonial governments, either acting on their own or carrying out royal decrees, established requirements that all farmers or all land owners plant some portion of their property in hemp. In one of its first decrees, for example, the Virginia Company required all Jamestown colonists in 1619 to set 100 cannabis plants and the governor to set an additional 5,000 plants. The Company also allotted 100 pounds to one Gabirel Wisher to hire men from Poland and Sweden to develop the hemp industry if they would emigrate to the new world (Abel 1982).

Similar laws sprung up throughout the colonies. For example, the General Court of Hartford in 1637 ordered all families in the colony to plant one teaspoon of hemp seed. The rationale behind this order, interestingly enough, was not to meet British needs, but to meet the growing demands for hemp products in the colonies "that we might in time have supply of linen cloth among ourselves," as the General Court order put it (as quoted in Nelson 2011, Chapter 2). Indeed, as with the Spanish, the English plan to install mammoth hemp plantations in the colonies to meet the needs of the home country failed. As the American colonies themselves began to grow and prosper, they found that they were able to make use of a large fraction of the hemp they produced, with relatively little to ship back to England. For example, by 1630, half of the colonial population was being clothed in hemp products grown on this side of the Atlantic (Booth 2005, 40).

Yet another European country with an interest in establishing hemp plantations in the New World was France. In 1606, the French explorer Samuel Champlain brought with him hemp seeds on his first trips to New France. There he assigned his botanist and apothecary, Louis Hébert, the task of determining how well the cannabis plant would grow in the new colony at Port Royal, Arcadia (now Nova Scotia). In fact, the French colonists were more concerned with growing enough food to survive, and hemp never became a favored crop in the French colonies (Abel 1982; also see Pickett and Pickett 2011, 164).

An ongoing question among historians is whether the cannabis plant was growing wild in North America when colonists first arrived in the first decade of the 17th century. By most accounts, it seems that it was. For example, the French explorer Jacques Cartier, reporting on his journeys to North America between 1535 and 1541, noted that "The land groweth fulle of Hempe which groweth of it selfe, which is as good as possibly may be seen, and as strong" (quoted in Nelson 2011). Other early explorers appeared to confirm this view. In 1719, for example, a Dutch farmer familiar with the cannabis plant reported on his visit to New Orleans that "hemp grows naturally on the lands adjoining to the lakes on the west of the

Mississippi. The stalks are as thick as one's finger, and about six feet long. They are quite like ours in the wood, the leaf and the rind" (quoted in Nelson 2011). Still, many modern observers believe that such judgments were inaccurate and that the plants reported as growing so abundantly were really other species, such as wood nettle (*Laportea canadensis*) or Indian hemp (*Apocynum cannabinum*).

In any case, there can be little doubt that the cannabis plant arrived in North America at a relatively early date and, perhaps more to the point, its intoxicating effects were well known to at least some cultures on the continent. For example, researchers have found stone and wooden pipes containing traces of cannabis dating back to 800 CE in the Ohio Valley (Bennett, Osburn, and Osburn 2001, 267–268). And some older members of Native American tribes recall their use of smoked cannabis in very old rituals (Spicer 2011).

The cannabis plant played an important role in American history in the three centuries following the foundation of the first colonies in Virginia and Massachusetts. In fact, American history is studded with interesting little facts about the role of both hemp and marijuana in American culture. For example, for a period of more than two centuries after the establishment of the Jamestown and Massachusetts Bay settlements, hemp was so widely grown and used that it was legal tender for payment of taxes and fines. For example, Virginia passed the Act for the Advancement of Manufactures in 1682, allowing the use of hemp, flax, wool, tar, and lumber, for the payment of taxes and other debts, with each product assigned a specific value per weight unit. In the case of hemp, that value was four pence per pound of hemp. Other colonies eventually passed similar laws—Maryland in 1706, Rhode Island in 1721, and Massachusetts in 1737—so that hemp remained a legal form of tender for well over a century (Nelson 2011, Chapter 2).

Some of the nation's leaders were so enamored of the plant that they either grew it themselves (George Washington and Thomas Jefferson) or used it in industries that they created

(Benjamin Franklin). In the latter case, Franklin, who was instrumental in the establishment of at least 18 new paper mills, arranged for one such mill to use hemp to produce paper, thus reducing the colonies' dependence on England for a supply of the paper it needed for books, documents, and other purposes (Nelson 2011, Chapter 2). When the War of Independence placed severe demand on the rapid production of new uniforms for the colonies' soldiers, wives, sisters, and daughters banded together to have spinning bees to make cloth for their soldier husbands, sons, and brothers ("Cannabis Comes to the New World" in Abel 1982).

The failure of the colonies to supply Mother England with the hemp it so desperately needed (see earlier discussion) eventually had historical significance in the relationship between the two countries. By the beginning of the 19th century, Russia had become the world's largest exporter of hemp, with neither England nor Spain nor, for that matter, the United States able to keep up with the demand for the product from their own domestic production. That imbalance of trade eventually had political consequences in 1807 with the signing of the Treaty of Tilset between Napoleon and Czar Alexander of Russia. One of the provisions of that treaty was that trade between Russia and England was no longer to be permitted. That provision was, of course, a disaster for England, which, at the time, was importing 90 percent of its hemp from Russia. As a way of getting around the provision, the English began commandeering American ships and crews, and sending them to Russia to purchase the hemp that the English needed. The controversy that developed over this issue between England and the United States eventually led to the outbreak of the War of 1812 (Herer 2001, Chapter 11).

As the United States developed after 1776, hemp production moved away from the East Coast, where it was replaced by more profitable crops, and began to develop in the Midwest. In particular, farms in Kentucky, Missouri, and Illinois began to supply the necessary hemp, primarily for the nation's sailing ships. The first hemp farms in the region were planted near Danville, Kentucky, in 1775, and their products were first advertised for sale 15 years later. Hemp was first grown in Missouri in 1835 and only five years later, the state was producing 12,500 tons of the product annually. The first hemp farms in Illinois were planted somewhat later, after 1875, while other hemp farms were also attempted in Nebraska, Indiana, Texas, and a few other states (Dvorak 2011). By 1870, the U.S. Census showed that the primary hemp-producing states were Kentucky (7,777 tons), Missouri (2,816 tons), and Tennessee (1,033 tons), with no other state producing more than 600 tons of the fiber (U.S. Bureau of the Census 1870, 85). The peak era for the production of hemp in the United States during the 19th century is probably the middle of the century. The U.S. Census for 1850 found that, at the time, there were 8,327 plantations growing hemp for cloth, canvas, cordage, and a variety of other purposes. The total value of the hemp crop for 1850 was said to be $5,247,480, making it the 18th most popular agricultural crop behind corn, wheat, cotton, hay, oats, potatoes, wool, tobacco, and a number of other products (U.S. Census 1854, 176).

In spite of these apparently promising beginnings, hemp farming never really became as successful in the United States as its adherents had hoped. Growing and harvesting hemp was a labor-intensive activity, and most farmers were barely able to make a living growing the crop. Over time, hemp was gradually replaced on most farms by more profitable crops such as cotton, jute, and sisal (Hemphasis 2011). Political and cultural factors also had their effects. Just prior to and during the Civil War, the Confederate Congress prohibited the exportation of cotton, negating the use of the hemp ropes that had been a major use for hemp being grown in the Midwest. This disturbance in the hemp market was not relieved by the end of the war, and hemp farming never really recovered its earlier heights or its proponents most enthusiastic expectations ("Cannabis Comes to the New World" in Abel 1982; Ehrensing 2011). By the end of the century, hemp farming had become a minor feature of the American agricultural industry, with the vast majority of the harvest being used to produce bird seed (still an important use of the product) and materials made from hemp seed oil, for example, varnish.

The hemp industry in Canada ultimately did no better than its cousin business in the United States. As noted earlier, Samuel Champlain tried to encourage the growth of hemp in the new French colony, but his hopes were not realized. His successors, usually with equal enthusiasm for a new hemp empire in Canada, met similar discouragement, as did the English when they took over the North American French colonies in 1763. The explanation for these failures was essentially the same as it was in the United States: farmers were simply not able to make a sufficient profit on hemp crops to justify the financial and labor costs of growing the crop. Even after a variety of appeals, including cash payments for raising the crop, grants of land on which to raise it, and appeals from church pulpits throughout the land, hemp farming continued to be a failure in Canada, as it was turning out to be in the United States ("Cannabis Comes to the New World," Abel 1982).

Hemp was not the only cannabis product that had reached the New World from Europe. Although its history is much different from that of hemp, marijuana also eventually became an important part of everyday life in the early United States during the mid-19th century. The impetus for that situation can be traced largely to the efforts of a single individual, the Irish physician William Brooke O'Shaughnessy. O'Shaughnessy served in India with the British East India Company from 1833 to 1841 and again from 1844 to 1860. While in India, he learned about the use of marijuana among native Indians for the treatment of a number of physical disorders. He attempted to formalize the use of marijuana for the treatment of his own patients by creating a variety of preparations and testing them on animals. He eventually became convinced of their value for the treatment of a variety of ailments, including pain and muscle spasms, as well as the vomiting and diarrhea associated with cholera that often led to a patient's death (O'Shaughnessy 1839; also see Mack and Joy 2001, 15–16).

O'Shaughnessey's research on marijuana interested and excited many of his colleagues, who designed and conducted their own experiments on the medical effects of the drug. Much of this research was summarized and analyzed toward the end of the century by a special committee appointed by the British government to study the reputed harmful effects of native Indians ingesting cannabis products. In their 1895 report, that committee, the India Hemp Drugs Commission, concluded that the use of hemp had no injurious physical, mental, or moral effects and that, in fact, it had a number of beneficial effects in the treatment of a variety of diseases and disorders (Young 1894).

The first medical conference in the United States devoted to the use of marijuana for medical purposes was held by the Ohio State Medical Society in 1860. The report of that meeting consists of a long list of personal testimonials by doctors who had had occasion to use the drug with patients or to perform experiments with the drug. Those reports covered a range from observations of frightening psychological events to almost miraculous cures of medical conditions that had been resistant to any other form of treatment (McMeens 1860).

Anecdotal reports from conferences like those of the Ohio State Medical Society were apparently sufficient to convince pharmaceutical companies to begin producing medications containing cannabis. Many histories of marijuana mention that some well-known pharmaceutical companies made available a variety of cannabis products beginning in the second half of the 19th century (e.g., Herer 2001). But the scope of that activity is difficult to envision. An invaluable source on this topic is the website *The Antique Cannabis Book*, which is a compendium of all known over-the-counter cannabis-containing medications available to the American public prior to adoption of the 1937 Marihuana Tax Act. The book lists more than 2,000 tinctures, extracts, home brews, corn remedies, antiasthmatic cigarettes, cough syrups, migraine headache products, veterinary medicines, prescription drugs, and other products. Photographs of the containers for most of these products are also available, providing a better explanation as to their contents and their intended uses. A review of this work makes it abundantly clear that the use of cannabis-related products in the period between 1850 and 1937 was not somewhat rare and unusual but, instead, was a common component of the collection of medicines for treating a host of disorders (Antique Cannabis Book 2011).

From the perspective of the early 21st century, it is sometimes difficult to realize the extent to which cannabis products permeated the American marketplace in the late 19th century. In his remarkable book *Cannabis: A History*, Martin Booth (2005) points out that cannabis products were widely recommended for use by married couples in the last half of the 19th century. One author, the "quack" doctor Frederick C. Hollis, for example, wrote a wildly popular (more than 200 editions) book, *The Marriage Guide; Or, Natural History of Generation: A Private Instructor for Married Persons and Those about to Marry*, in which he encouraged readers to order from him an aphrodisiac in which hashish was a constituent (Booth 2005, 120–121). Perhaps most ironic of all was the effort by some members of the Women's Temperance Movement in the late 1800s to encourage men to replace their consumption of alcohol with the use of marijuana. The basis for this campaign was the belief that men would be less likely to abuse their wives and girlfriends if they were under the influence of marijuana rather than under the influence of alcohol (Booth 2005, 121).

Cannabis was present in a number of seemingly less innocuous products also. For example, beginning in the 1860s, the Gunjah Wallah Company of New York City began producing a "hasheesh candy" that it called The Arabian "Gunja" of Enchantment, which was a confectionized preparation of cannabis. Advertisements for the candy claimed that it was a "most pleasurable and harmless stimulant" that cured a number of medical conditions, including nervousness, weakness, and melancholy. It also "inspire[d] all classes with new life and energy" and acted as "a complete mental and physical invigorator" (Maple Sugar Hashish Candy 2011). Whatever appeals cannabis products may have had as patent medicines, tonics, marriage aphrodisiacs, or confectionary products, the greatest official public attention was always paid to hemp as an agricultural product. And statistical evidence suggests that that product had become a minor component of American agriculture by the end of the 19th century. As Table 1.2 shows, the amount of land devoted to hemp farming in the United States and the total amount of hemp produced remained relatively constant, and relatively small, from the last

Table 1.2   Acreage Devoted to Hemp Farming and Hemp Production, 1876–1940

Period	Acreage	Production (in tons)
1876–1880	15,000	7,000
1881–1885	11,000	5,000
1886–1890	16,000	7,500
1891–1895	11,000	5,000
1896–1900	10,000	4,500
1901–1905	12,000	5,500
1906–1910	10,000	4,500
1911–1913	10,000	4,500
1914–1918	10,500	8,500
1919–1923	8,600	3,800
1924–1928	4,300	1,800
1929–1933	1,200	500
1934–1938	7,100	600
1940	241	(no record)

Source: West, David P. "Industrial Hemp Farming: History and Practice." http://www.gametec.com/hemp/IndHmpFrmg.htm. West's data were apparently derived from J. Merritt Matthews and Herbert R. Mauersberger. *Matthews' Textile Fibers: Their Physical, Microscopical, and Chemical Properties (5th ed.)*. New York: J. Wiley & Sons, 1947, which, in turn, apparently obtained its data from a U.S. Department of Agriculture Bulletin, "Hemp, Its Production and Use as a Fiber Crop," date unknown.

quarter of the 19th century to 1937, when the Marihuana Tax Act (see Chapter 2) was passed. For most of the 20th century, then, hemp farming was a largely insignificant component of the U.S. agricultural system.

For all intents and purposes, adoption of the Marihuana Tax Act of 1937 brought to an end the agricultural production of hemp in the United States. Although that act was aimed primarily at reducing the availability of marijuana as a recreational drug in the country, a side effect was the prohibition on the growing of cannabis plants that had any THC at all in them, and that included hemp plants. Even though the level of THC in hemp plants is very low (usually much less than 1 percent), it is not zero. This provision of the act accounts for the production of hemp in the country dropping to less than 250 tons by 1940.

World War II, however, created a challenge for the U.S. government with regard to the growing of hemp. A number of products important to the war effort, for example, sail canvas, rope, and military uniforms, had previously been made from imported hemp or other fibers from countries now occupied by the Japanese. To compensate for the loss of these fibers, the U.S. government decided to provide waivers from the 1937 act for farmers who were willing to start growing hemp again to meet wartime needs. In 1942, the U.S. Department of Agriculture (USDA) made a film, *Hemp for Victory*, extolling the virtues of hemp as a farm crop and encouraging American farmers to start growing the crop as their contribution to the war effort. (The USDA and Library of Congress later denied that such a film was ever made, although they reversed that view when copies of the film were later donated to the library.) The film is in the public domain and can be viewed at a number of Internet sites (e.g., see "Hemp for Victory" (1942); http://www.archive.org/details/Hemp_for_victory_1942).

The USDA campaign to increase hemp production was successful, with a huge upswing in the amount of land planted with the crop; the amount of hemp produced peaked during the

Table 1.3   Hemp Production in the United States, 1931–1946

Year	Acreage	Production (long tons)
1931	320	122
1932	200	71
1933	140	47
1934	500	190
1935	700	273
1936	1,400	453
1937	1,300	465
1938	1,390	556
1939	1,440	572
1940	2,070	738
1941	7,400	3,308
1942	14,500	6,216
1943	146,200	62,803
1944	68,200	30,130
1945	6,500	2,232
1946	4,800	1,715

Source: Ash, Anne L. 1948. "Hemp: Production and Utilization." *Economic Botany* 2: 158–169. Data for this article was taken from U.S. Department of Agriculture. *Agricultural Statistics*. Washington, DC: Government Printing Office, 1945.

middle of the war (see Table 1.3). However, the end of the war saw the reimposition of federal controls on the planting and harvesting of hemp, and production dropped essentially to zero over the following half century ("Industrial Hemp Profile" 2011). A small hemp industry was maintained in Wisconsin until 1958, when it too was abandoned. ("Industrial Hemp in the United States" 2011). In response to pressure from producers of hemp products, however, that trend may now be starting to change. In 2002, Hawaii became the first state to license the planting and harvesting of hemp under strict, federally approved regulations. Over the next decade, 23 states began negotiations with the federal government for permission to grow hemp crops, and 14 of those states have taken legislative action formally requesting such approval ("Industrial Hemp Profile" 2011; Johnson 2010). An era of hemp production may have returned to the United States.

Although currently banned in the United States, the production of hemp is legal in some other parts of the world. As of early 2012, the crop may be grown in about 30 countries worldwide, including Australia, Austria, Canada, Chile, China, France, Great Britain, North Korea, Russia, and Spain. Some of these countries never banned the growing and harvesting of hemp products, while others had such a ban at one time in the past, but have since revoked it (Johnson 2011). According to the latest data available from the UN Food and Agriculture Organization (FAO), the largest producer of hemp fiber in the world is China (44,000 tonnes in 2009), followed by North Korea (13,000 tonnes), Chile (4,388 tonnes), Romania (3,000 tonnes), and Russia (1,500 tonnes). China also leads the world in the production of hempseed with a harvest of 48,000 tonnes in 2009, followed by France (6,971 tonnes), Chile (1,220 tonnes), Ukrakine (842 tonnes), and Hungary (583 tonnes) (FAOSTAT 2011).

In Conclusion

This chapter has shown that humans have known about and grown the cannabis plant for more than 5,000 years. They have found a variety of uses for the plant, including the manufacture of clothing, sails, rope, and oils, as well as its inclusion in religious and ceremonial occasions. It has also been used by many cultures for many different medical applications. Finally, in the form of marijuana and hashish, humans have used the cannabis plant for recreational purposes. The United States as well as other nations and governmental units have banned some or all of these uses at one or another time in history. Over the centuries, the cannabis plant has gone from being a highly respected sometimes holy object of veneration to one that is viewed with the greatest opprobrium by some cultures. Chapter 2 provides a review of how this dramatic change came about and the issues the change has raised in modern societies around the world.

Note

Introduction

The literature dealing with marijuana contains a large number of interesting little facts about cannabis that are repeated on many websites and in many print references. The statement that "Chinese Emperor Shen-Nung prescribed cannabis for a variety of ailments as early as 2737 BCE" is an example of such a fact. The author has attempted to locate a primary source for each of these interesting little facts included in this book, sometimes successfully, sometimes not. The reader should be aware that simple repetition of a statement in many references does not constitute proof that that statement is true and that any secondary citation provided here (or in any other reference) is inherently subject to some level of uncertainty.

References

738 F.2d 497: *United States of America, Appellee, v. Donald Nixon Rush, Larry Joseph Lancelotti, Gregory Leelancelotti, Harry J. Shnurman, Robert Michael Cohen, Thomasg. Converse, David Earl Johnson, Irving F. Imoberstag, Carleric Olsen, Jacob Shnurman, Randall Collins, Jeffrey Allenbrown, and David Nissenbaum, Defendants; Appellants, United States of America, Appellee, v. Michael Lee Risolvato, Defendant; Appellants, United States of America, Appellee, v. Charles Leaton, Defendant, Appellant.* http://law.justia.com/cases/federal/appellate-courts/F2/738/497/135233/. Accessed on December 19, 2011.

"98 Percent Of All Domestically Eradicated Marijuana Is 'Ditchweed,' DEA Admits." NORML. http://norml.org/news/2006/09/07/98-percent-of-all-domestically-eradicated-marijuana-is-ditchweed-dea-admits. Accessed on December 16, 2011.

Abel, Ernest L. 1982. *Marijuana: The First Twelve Thousand Years.* New York: McGraw Hill. Available online at http://

www.druglibrary.org/schaffer/hemp/history/first12000/abel. htm. Accessed on December 18, 2011.

"Antique Cannabis Book." http://antiquecannabisbook.com/. Accessed on December 22, 2011.

Balfour, Edward Green. 1873. *The Cyclopaedia of India and of Eastern and Southern Asia, Commercial, Industrial, and Scientific: Products of the Mineral, Vegetable, and Animal Kingdoms, Useful Arts and Manufactures* (2nd ed.). London: B. Quaritch.

Benet, Sula. 1975. "Early Diffusion and Folk Uses of Hemp." In Rubin, Vera, ed., *Cannabis and Culture.* The Hague: Mouton, 39–49. Also available online at http://khem-caigan .livejournal.com/3259.html.

Bennett, Chris, Lynn Osburn, and Judith Osburn. 2001. *Green Gold: Marijuana in Magic and Religion.* Frazier Park, CA: Access Unlimited.

Booth, Martin. 2005. *Cannabis: A History.* New York: Picador Press.

Brecher, Edward M., and the Editors of Consumer Reports. 1972. *Licit and Illicit Drugs.* Mount Vernon, NY: Consumers Union.

"Cannabis/Marijuana (Δ^9-Tetrahydrocannabinol, THC)." Drugs and Human Performance Fact Sheets. http://www .nhtsa.gov/People/injury/research/job185drugs/cannabis .htm. Accessed on December 16, 2011.

"Cesamet." RxList. http://www.rxlist.com/cesamet-drug.htm. Accessed on December 16, 2011.

Creighton, C. 1903. "On Indications of the Hachish-Vice in the Old Testament." *JANUS, Archives Internationales pour l'Histoire de la Medecine et la Geographie Medicale, Huitieme Annee.* 241–246. Cited in http://www.erowid.org/plants/ cannabis/cannabis_spirit4.shtml. Accessed on December 19, 2011.

"DEA Clarifies Status of Hemp in the Federal Register." U.S. Drug Enforcement Administration. http://www.justice.gov/ dea/pubs/pressrel/pr100901.html. Accessed on December 16, 2011.

"Definitions and Explanations." http://www.cannabis-med.org/ science/science-definitions.htm. Accessed on December 16, 2011.

Deitch, Robert. 2003. *Hemp: American History Revisited: The Plant with a Divided History.* New York: Algora Publishing.

Dvorak, John. "America's Harried Hemp History." http:// www.hemphasis.net/History/harriedhemp.htm. Accessed on December 22, 2011.

Ehrensing, Daryl T. "Feasibility of Industrial Hemp Production in the United States Pacific Northwest." http://extension .oregonstate.edu/catalog/html/sb/sb681/#History. Accessed on December 22, 2011.

Emboden, William A. Jr. 1972. "Ritual Use of Cannabis Sativa L." In Furst, Peter T., ed., *Flesh of the Gods.* New York: Praeger.

Ethiopian Zion Coptic Church. 1988. *Marijuana and the Bible.* Boston: Beacon Press. Available online at http://www .erowid.org/plants/cannabis/cannabis_spirit2.shtml. Accessed on December 19, 2011.

FAOSTAT. Food and Agriculture Organization of the United Nations. http://faostat.fao.org/DesktopDefault.aspx? PageID=567#ancor. Accessed on December 24, 2011.

"The First Anaesthetic in the World: Mafei San." Safedom.net. http://english.safedom.net/pedia/41.html. Accessed on December 18, 2011.

Fleming, M. P., and R. C. Clarke. 1998. "Physical Evidence for the Antiquity of Cannabis Sativa L. (Cannabaceae)." *Journal of the International Hemp Association* 5(2), 80–92.

Freeman, Brian C., and Gwyn A. Beattie. "An Overview of Plant Defenses against Pathogens and Herbivores." APSnet.

http://www.apsnet.org/edcenter/intropp/topics/Pages/Overview
OfPlantDiseases.aspx. Accessed on December 16, 2011.

González, Gustavo. "Marijuana's Virtues Cast in Doubt."
Tierramérica. http://www.tierramerica.net/2003/0119/
iarticulo.shtml. Accessed on December 21, 2011.

Goodman, Jordan, Paul E Lovejoy, and Andrew Sherratt. 2007.
*Consuming Habits: Global and Historical Perspectives on How
Cultures Define Drugs* (2nd ed.). London; New York: Routledge.

Gumbiner, Jann. "History of Cannabis in India." Psychology
Today. http://www.psychologytoday.com/blog/the-teenage-
mind/201106/history-cannabis-in-india. Accessed on
December 18, 2011.

Hanuš, Lumir, and Raphael Mechoulam. 2008. "The
Chemistry of Major New Players in Physiology." In Ikan,
Raphael, ed., *Selected Topics in the Chemistry of Natural
Products*. Singapore: World Scientific.

"Hasish." Drugs.com. http://www.drugs.com/hashish.html.
Accessed on December 18, 2011.

"Hashish and the Arabs." Schaffer Library of Drug Policy.
http://druglibrary.org/schaffer/hemp/history/first12000/2
.htm. Accessed on September 30, 2012.

"The Hashish Club." FriendsOfCannabis.com. http://www
.friendsofcannabis.com/directory/index.php?option=com_
alphacontent&section=18&Itemid=58&cat=338. Accessed
on December 21, 2011.

"Hashish History." The Vaults of Erowid. http://www.erowid
.org/plants/cannabis/cannabis_history_hashish.shtml.
Accessed on December 21, 2011.

"Hemphasis." http://www.hemphasis.net/History/history.htm.
Accessed on December 22, 2011.

Herer, Jack. 2001. *The Emperor Wears No Clothes* (11th ed.).
Anaheim, CA: AH HA Publishing. Also available online at
http://www.jackherer.com/thebook/.

"History of Hemp Fibre." http://www.midrealm.org/starleafgate/ pdf/Hemp_Fibre.pdf. Accessed on October 1, 2012.

"Industrial Hemp in the United States: Status and Market Potential." Economic Research Service, U.S. Department of Agriculture. http://www.ers.usda.gov/publications/ ages001E/ages001E.pdf. Accessed on December 24, 2011.

"Industrial Hemp Profile." Agricultural Marketing Resource Center. http://www.agmrc.org/commodities__products/ fiber/industrial_hemp_profile.cfm. Accessed on December 24, 2011.

"Information on Acomplia® (Rimonabant) (Possibly Zimulti®). CB1 Cannabinoid Receptor Antagonist." http:// www.rimonabant-information.com/. Accessed on December 16, 2011.

Johnson, Renée. *Hemp as an Agricultural Commodity.* Congressional Research Service, December 22, 2010. http:// www.nationalaglawcenter.org/assets/crs/RL32725.pdf. Accessed on December 24, 2011.

Li, Hui-Lin. 1974a. "An Archaeological and Historical Account of Cannabis in China." *Economic Botany* 28(4), 437–48.

Li, Hui-Lin. 1974b. "The Origin and Use of Cannabis in Eastern Asia Linguistic-Cultural Implications." *Economic Botany* 28(3): 293–301.

Lu, Xiaozhai, and Robert C. Clarke. 1995. "The Cultivation and Use of Hemp *(Cannabis Sativa L.)* in Ancient China." *Journal of the International Hemp Association* 2(1): 26–30. Archived online at http://www.internationalhempassociation.org/jiha/ iha02111.html.

Mack, Alison, and Janet Joy. 2000. *Marijuana as Medicine: The Science beyond Controversy.* Washington, D.C.: National Academies Press.

"Maple Sugar Hashish Candy." ElectricEmperor.com. http:// www.electricemperor.com/eecdrom/HTML/EMP/12/ ECH12_03.HTM. Accessed on December 23, 2011.

"Marinol." RxList. http://www.rxlist.com/marinol-drug.htm. Accessed on December 16, 2011.

McMeens, R. R. 1860. "Report of the Ohio State Medical Committee on Cannabis Indica." *Transactions of the Fifteenth Annual Meeting of the Ohio State Medical Society at Ohio White Sulphur Springs*, June 12 to 14, 1860, pp. 75–100. Available online at http://www.onlinepot.org/medical/Dr_ Tods_PDFs/s3_1.pdf.

Menelik, Girma Yohannes Iyassu. 2009. *Rastafarians: A Movement Tied with a [sic] Social and Psychological Conflicts.* [Munich]: GRIN. Verlag.

Merlin, M. D. 2003. "Archaeological Evidence for the Tradition of Psychoactive Plant Use in the Old World." *Economic Botany* 57(3): 295–323.

Nelson, Robert A. *A History of Hemp*. http://www.rexresearch .com/hhist/hhicon.htm. Accessed December 21, 2011.

Oner, S. T., ed. 2011. *Cannabis Indica: The Essential Guide to the World's Finest Marijuana Strains*. San Francisco: Green Candy Press.

O'Shaughnessy, W. B. "On the Preparations Of the Indian Hemp, or Gunjah *(Cannabis Indica)*; Their Effects on the Animal System in Health, and Their Utility in the Treatment of Tetanus and Other Convulsive Diseases" (originally published in 1839). In Tod H. Mikuriya, *Marijuana Medical Papers (1839–1972)*. Oakland, CA: Medi-Comp Press, 1973. Also available online at http://www.marijuanalibrary .org/Dr_Mikuriya.html.

Pickett, Margaret F., and Dwayne W. Pickett. 2011. *The European Struggle to Settle North America: Colonizing Attempts by England, France and Spain, 1521–1608*. Jefferson, NC: McFarland & Company.

Rabelais, Master Francis. 1894. *Five Books of the Lives, Heroic Deeds and Sayings of Gargantua and His Son Pantagruel*. Derby, UK: Moray Press. Project Gutenberg. http://www

.gutenberg.org/files/1200/1200-h/p3.htm. Accessed on
December 20, 2011.

Rudgley, Richard. "Cannabis." *Encyclopedia of Psychoactive
Substances*. http://cannabis.net/hist/index.html. Accessed on
December 18, 2011.

1 Samuel 14 (New International Version). BibleGateway.com.
http://www.biblegateway.com/passage/?search=1+Samuel
+14&version=NIV. Accessed on December 19, 2011.

Shrank, Cathy. "Bullein's Bulwark" (originally, in full: *Bullein's
Bulwark of Defence against all Sickness, Soreness, and Wounds
that dooe daily assault Mankinde*). http://www.hrionline.ac
.uk/origins/DisplayServlet?id=Bullein4033&type=normal.
Accessed on December 20, 2011.

Smith, Frederick Porter. 1911. *Chinese Materia Medica:
Vegetable Kingdom*. Shanghai: American Presbyterian
Mission Press. Available online at http://www.archive.org/
stream/chinesemateriame00stuauoft/chinesemateriame00
stuauoft_djvu.txt.

"Sourcebook of Criminal Justice Statistics Online." http://
www.albany.edu/sourcebook/pdf/t4382005.pdf. Accessed
on December 16, 2011.

Spicer, Leah. *Historical and Cultural Uses of Cannabis and the
Canadian "Marijuana Clash."* Report prepared for the Senate
Special Committee on Illegal Drugs. http://www.parl.gc.ca/
Content/SEN/Committee/371/ille/library/spicer-e.htm#2.
Central Asia. Accessed on December 18, 2011.

Stafford, Ned. "Synthetic Cannabis Mimic Found in Herbal
Incense." Cannabis Culture. http://www.cannabisculture
.com/v2/news/synthetic-cannabis-mimic-found-in-herbal-
incense. Accessed on December 16, 2011.

Stanley, Alessandra. "Moscow Journal; Tattooed Lady, 2,000
Years Old, Blooms Again." *New York Times*, July 13, 1994.
Also available online at http://www.nytimes.com/1994/07/

13/world/moscow-journal-tattooed-lady-2000-years-old-blooms-again.html. Accessed on December 18, 2011.

Stefanis, C., C. Ballas, and D. Madianou. 1975. "Sociocultural and Epidemiological Aspects of Hashish Use in Greece." In Rubin, Vera, ed., *Cannabis and Culture.* The Hague: Mouton, 303–326.

U.S. Bureau of the Census. *The Statistics of the Wealth and Industry of the United States.* Washington, DC: Government Printing Office, 1870. Available online at http://www2.census.gov/prod2/decennial/documents/1870c-02.pdf.

U.S. Census. *Statistical View of the United States.* Washington, DC: Beverley Tucker, Senate Printer, 1854. Available online at http://www2.census.gov/prod2/decennial/documents/1850c-06.pdf

Weiss, Brian L. [Summary of psychiatric examination of Ethiopian Zion Coptic Church members]. 1980. http://www.ethiopianzioncopticchurch.org/Agency/amicus_19880713_ex07.pdf. Accessed on December 19, 2011.

West, David P. "Industrial Hemp Farming: History and Practice." http://www.gametec.com/hemp/IndHmpFrmg.htm. Accessed on December 23, 2011.

Young, W. Mackworth et al. 1894. *Report of the Indian Hemp Drugs Commission, 1893–94.* [n.p.]: Government Central Printing Office, vol. 1, 263–264. Also available online at http://www.drugtext.org/Table/Indian-Hemp-Commission-Report/.

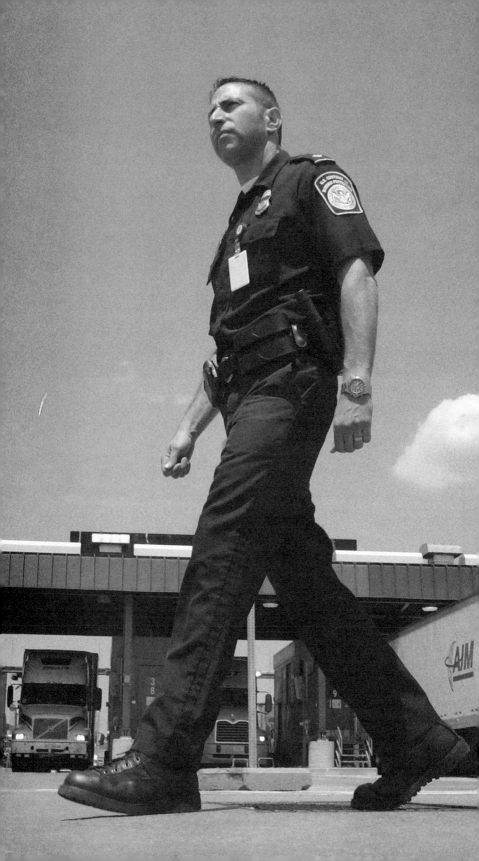

2   Problems, Controversies, and Solutions

The inspection was expected to be routine. For years, the Canadian company, Kenex, Ltd., had been shipping hemp seed to the Nutiva company in Sebastopol, California, for use in its bird seed. Jean Laprise, the president of Kenex, expected the present shipment of hemp seed to clear customs at the U.S. border without any problems. So Mr. Laprise was a bit shocked, to say the least, when U.S. custom agents impounded all 40,000 pounds of hemp seed and shipped them for storage in a Detroit, Michigan, warehouse. The hemp seed contained THC, custom agents said, so it could not be admitted to the United States under a provision of the 1970 Controlled Substances Act (CSA). The news was a surprise to Mr. Laprise at least in part because hemp growers in Canada have long been scrupulous in ensuring that their products contain a very low level of THC, always less than 1 percent. The hemp seed in question had been analyzed and was found to contain about 0.0014 percent, not enough, according to one observer, to "give a bird a buzz" (Wren 2011). What was the logic behind the decision to impound a legitimate agricultural product from Canada that has such a modest likelihood of being used as an illegal drug in the

---

Importation of any amount of a controlled substance, such as cannabis, into the United States can be punished by a cash fine and/or imprisonment for a period of up to five years. (AP Photo/David Duprey)

United States? (For additional examples of the U.S. campaign against hemp products, also see Barnett 2011; Bonné 2011.)

History of Cannabis Prohibition

Throughout history, humans have had a profound love/hate relationship with the cannabis plant. On the one hand, it has provided a host of valuable materials in the form of hemp, which has been used for cloth, twine, rope, cordage, sails, yarn, body-care products, paper, pet foods, hemp seed oil, and, of course, bird seed. In the form of marijuana and hashish, it has provided a gateway to out-of-body experiences that have been understood as a simple "high"—an escape from the often less-than-pleasant humdrum of everyday life—or a window to the sacred. But many cultures have also viewed such experiences as too much of an escape from reality, too much like the tale of Icarus, who flew too far from Earth's surface and too close to the heavenly orb, losing his life in the process. And so, the history of *Cannabis sativa* is as much a story of caution, risk, and prohibition as it is of anything else.

Should the use of cannabis by humans be prohibited? If so, which forms of the plant and under what circumstances? These questions are as controversial in the early 21st century as it has been throughout human history. Some people argue that the choice of using or not using hemp, marijuana, and/or hashish is one that should be left to individuals; governments have no authority to prohibit the use of a plant that humans have used safely for millennia. Others are more cautious in their views, suggesting that hemp is certainly a harmless and valuable material, although other forms of cannabis are more problematic. Still others see useful applications of marijuana as a therapeutic agent, although its uses as a recreational drug pose more difficult issues. Finally, other individuals argue that the cannabis plant poses such great dangers—even to birds—that all forms should be banned under all circumstances. Understanding historical attitudes about prohibitions on the use of cannabis provides a perspective from which to understand today's debate about the plant.

Prohibitions on Cannabis: Ancient Cultures

Throughout most of human history, the use of cannabis products has not been a matter of controversy. Hemp has long been almost universally considered a valuable material for making a host of useful products. And healers of all kinds—from shamans to modern physicians—have commonly turned to marijuana as an important tool in their materia medica. Even the use of marijuana to achieve out-of-body experiences, as is done in religious ceremonies, has generally been more widely praised than condemned. In spite of this generally positive view of the cannabis plant, there have always been cultures in which negative attitudes outweighed positive beliefs, and the plant fell into disrepute among leaders of the society and/or the general public.

As an example, some historians believe that acceptance and/ or tolerance for the use of marijuana in achieving psychoactive effects began to wane in China during the Han dynasty (206 BCE–220 CE) largely because Chinese society was developing a more rational outlook on life and saw a consequent reduction in dependence on shamanism (and hence, on psychoactive drugs). This change eventually resulted in the view that marijuana was a "disreputable" herb not worthy of use by true healers (Touw 1981, 23). Early Islamists also seem to have taken a somewhat neutral view toward cannabis since it was apparently not specifically prohibited in the Quran. Indeed, in view of the Prophet's specific prohibition of the use of alcohol, the use of cannabis seems to have become at first the psychoactive drug of choice within early Islamic society. That situation changed over time, however, as more and more scholars adopted the view that the traditional Quranic prohibition of *khamr* (literally, "fermented grape") referred not only to alcoholic beverages, but also to any substance that "befogs the mind" ("Alcohol and Intoxicants in Islam" 2012). That interpretation obviously added cannabis to the list of substances forbidden to believers in Islam. The controversy over the true interpretation of khamr and the implication of that interpretation remains a matter of some controversy today (see, for example, "Is Marijuana Haram?" 2012). In spite of the Islamic position, however, cannabis appears far more likely to have been viewed as a beneficial (or, at least, a harmless) natural product until the early 20th century. Its worst effects generally seemed to be seen as erratic behavior when used in excess, especially by mentally unstable individuals already predisposed to antisocial actions.

International Concerns, 1910–1925

The casual acceptance of cannabis began to change significantly during the first two decades of the 20th century, when the world began to consider the potentially harmful (to individuals) and dangerous (to society) consequences of narcotic abuse, especially from derivatives of the coca plant (cocaine) and opiates such as opium and heroin. Similar fears about the risks and dangers of other drugs, such as alcohol, nicotine (tobacco), and caffeine (coffee) had largely run their course before the end of the 19th century. Such concerns had led to the bans, among many possible examples, on the drinking of coffee in Egypt in 1524, and on the use of tobacco throughout Christendom in 1624 (Hanauer and Pickthall 2007, 291–292; Christen, Swanson, Glover, and Henderson 1982, 825).

The first international meeting called to discuss and act on the (perceived) rising threat of narcotic drugs was the International Opium Commission, held in Shanghai in 1909. That meeting was held at the instigation of the U.S. government and was attended by representatives from 12 nations in addition to the United States: Austria-Hungary, China, France, Germany, Italy, Japan, Netherlands, Persia (now Iran), Portugal, Russia, Siam (now Thailand), and the United Kingdom. The meeting was careful not to call itself a conference, which would have permitted the drafting and signing of an official international treaty. It did, however, unanimously adopt a statement of principle in opposition to the trade of opium products among nations of the world ("The Shanghai Opium Commission" 2012).

One of the recommendations produced at the Shanghai meeting was that a follow-up conference be held to further consider the problem of narcotics trade and use around the world. That meeting was held in The Hague in 1912. It was chaired by Bishop Charles Henry Brent of the United States, who had also chaired the Shanghai meeting. Attendees included the same nations that had assembled in Shanghai, except for Austria-Hungary. The treaty entered into force two years later in five countries: China, Honduras, the Netherlands, Norway, and the United States. In 1919, the treaty received much wider acceptance when it became part of the Treaty of Versailles, which ended World War I. At that point, it took effect in 60 nations worldwide. The United States remained a signatory to the original Hague treaty, although it was not then (and never was) a member of the League of Nations, under which the treaty was administered.

An effort to include cannabis in the Hague Treaty had been made by the United States, which suggested that it be included among the narcotic drugs for which information would be exchanged among signatories to the treaty (Marijuana is not a narcotic, but it has long been so labeled, especially by individuals and organizations that support increased control over its sale and use). That proposal was rejected, however, as other members of the convention were not convinced that there was as yet enough information about the risks posed by cannabis or its use throughout the world. They did agree, however, to recommend that additional research be conducted on cannabis with a view to reconsider the U.S. recommendation at a later date. That research was never actually carried out ("The Cannabis Problem" 2012).

Cannabis finally received attention as a potentially harmful and dangerous drug at the international level just prior to the 1925 International Convention on Narcotics Control, sponsored by the League of Nations and held in Geneva, Switzerland. The subject of marijuana—then commonly known as *Indian hemp*—was raised by delegates from Egypt and Turkey, who told spine-tingling tales of the disastrous consequences of its use in their countries. The Egyptian delegate, Dr. Mohamed Abdel Salam El Guindy, for example, claimed that the use of hashish was responsible for most of the cases of insanity occurring his country. He described the typical cannabis user as follows:

> His eye is wild and the expression of his face is stupid. He is silent; has no muscular power; suffers from physical ailments, heart troubles, digestive troubles etc; his intellectual faculties gradually weaken and the whole organism decays. The addict very frequently becomes neurasthenic and eventually insane. (cited in United Nations Office on Drugs and Crime 2010, 54; also see Kendell 2003, 144–145)

Warnings such as these carried the day among the Geneva delegates, and they devoted two chapters of the final treaty (IV and V) to recommending a ban on all uses of cannabis except for medical and scientific uses, which were not defined. The actual claims about the effects of cannabis put forward by Dr. El Guindy—which differed dramatically from those contained in the report of the 1893 Indian Hemp Drugs Commission Report—were not investigated before the Geneva delegates adopted the final treaty. The United States never signed the Geneva Convention because it was not a member of the League at the time, and also because U.S. delegates thought that the conference's attitudes about and approach to the control of dangerous drugs was too lenient, certainly more lenient than policies then being developed at home.

Prohibition of Cannabis: The United States

Indeed, by the first decade of the 20th century, a number of U.S. politicians, law enforcement officials, social reformers, and members of the general public had become convinced that mind-altering drugs of all kinds posed a severe danger, not only to the individuals who used them, but far more importantly, to the stability of society itself. These individuals and the organizations they founded and/or represented were instrumental not only in calling the Shanghai and Hague meetings, but also, ultimately, in the adoption of the 18th Amendment to the U.S. Constitution, prohibiting the sale of alcohol, in 1919, and adoption of the Harrison Narcotics Act of 1914, which established a tax on producing, manufacturing, compounding, importing, distributing, and selling cocaine in the United States. And although the first federal law limiting the use of cannabis in the United States was not passed until 1937, a movement to label the drug as a dangerous narcotic had been well under way many years earlier. That movement did not develop in a vacuum in the United States but, instead, was deeply associated with a more general cultural trend toward the prohibition of any type of mind-altering substance. In their classic analysis of the process by which marijuana use was criminalized in the United States, Bonnie and Whitebread (1970) have pointed out that

at each stage of its development marijuana policy has been heavily influenced by other social issues because the drug has generally been linked with broader cultural patterns. . . . In fact, the facility with which marijuana policy was initiated directly related to the astoundingly sudden and extreme alteration of public narcotics and alcohol policy between 1900 and 1920. (Bonnie and Whitebread 1970, Chapter 3)

Until the 1930s, concerns about the risks posed by "dangerous drugs" in the United States—as in the rest of the world—focused almost entirely on cocaine and opiates; cannabis was rarely mentioned. In the United States, marijuana was not mentioned in any federal drug legislation until the Uniform Narcotics Drug Act was adopted in 1932. That act encouraged individual states to bring their drug laws into agreement with the 1922 Narcotic Drug Import and Export Law, which had placed restrictions on the distribution of cocaine and opiates (cannabis was not mentioned in the act). At the time, state drug laws differed widely from each other and from the restrictions included in the Narcotic Drug Import and Export law. One of the provisions of the 1932 act dealt with cannabis, including it with cocaine and opiates, a provision that had not been included in the 1922 act. No explanation was given in the act as to the reason for this broadening, and the act was adopted with the addition of cannabis (Bonnie and Whitebread 1970, Chapter 4). The legal status of cannabis at the state level during the first three decades of the 20th century was different from that at the national level. As early as 1913, some local communities and states had begun to adopt legislation criminalizing the growing, distribution, and/or use of cannabis products. What were the forces, Bonnie and Whitebread (1970) have asked, that motivated this trend toward the criminalization of marijuana, a trend that eventually became an aggressive national movement by the 1930s?

Their research points to three such factors: class and racial prejudices; concerns that drug users would switch from more tightly controlled drugs like cocaine and heroin to marijuana (the theory of "substitution"); and an international trend toward the criminalization of marijuana, as expressed in the 1912 Hague Convention and the 1925 Geneva Convention (Bonnie and Whitebread 1970, Chapter 3). Bonnie and Whitebread point out that the earliest laws criminalizing the use of marijuana were passed in the western states at a time when Mexican immigration was increasing dramatically, largely because of the number of Mexican nationals who were fleeing the revolution of 1910 through 1920. At the time, marijuana was used almost exclusively by these immigrants, and that practice was quickly associated with a generally agreed upon perception that Mexicans were poorly educated and of low moral character. Their use of marijuana as a recreational drug was, ipso facto, an indication of the risks it posed. Bonnie and Whitebread provide a number of specific examples in which states passed anticannabis laws based on clearly racist views with little or no public debate, or even thoughtful discussion within legislatures. They cite a newspaper report of the debate in the Montana legislature in 1929 over criminalizing marijuana use. One legislator noted that a Mexican who has smoked marijuana "thinks he has just been elected president of Mexico so he starts out to execute all his political enemies." In response, "[e]verybody laughed and the bill was recommended for passage" (Bonnie and Whitebread 1970, Chapter 3). Based on the many examples they found, Bonnie and Whitebread concluded that "legislative action and approval [of anticannabis laws] were essentially kneejerk responses uninformed by scientific study or public debate and colored instead by racial bias and sensationalistic myths" (Bonnie and Whitebread 1970, Chapter 3). In any case, laws prohibiting the sale of marijuana swept through the United States between 1914 and 1931, with 26 states including some form of prohibition in their laws.

Such laws were not restricted to the western states, although the motivation for laws in the East was considerably different from those in the West. The most common basis for anticannabis laws in the East, Bonnie and Whitebread (1970) found, was fear that marijuana use would grow if laws related to cocaine and opiates were tightened (as was occurring at the time). The argument is one that is still heard today, namely that drug users will switch to a new drug (such as marijuana) as other drugs (such as cocaine and heroin) are more tightly controlled. This philosophy, Bonnie and Whitebread believe, was the primary basis for anticannabis laws passed in Maine, Massachusetts, Michigan, New York, Ohio, Rhode Island, and Vermont in the period between 1914 and 1947. For example, when New York City added marijuana to its list of prohibited drugs in 1914, the *New York Times* commented that users of cannabis "are now hardly numerous enough to count, but they are likely to increase as other narcotics become harder to obtain" ("Sanitary Code Adjustments" 1914, 8).

Cannabis Legislation in the States

Legislators in the United States awakened to the (supposed) threat posed by cannabis began looking for ways of dealing with this new problem as early as the 1910s. Those efforts took two general approaches: taxation on the production, distribution, and (less commonly) use of marijuana, as a way of reducing demand for the drug, and outright bans on cannabis in any and all forms. The federal government was relatively timid in acting on the cannabis problem, not passing the first national law on the drug until 1937. A number of local communities and states, however, had begun to take action against cannabis much earlier. The first state law prohibiting the use of marijuana was adopted in California in 1913. The law was actually a technical amendment to the state's poison laws, proposed by the state's Board of Pharmacy. It was apparently inspired by concerns over the use of narcotic drugs by the state's Chinese residents (Gieringer 1999, 2). The law received essentially no public attention at the time; historians often pass it over and point to a law adopted in Utah in 1915 as the first state law dealing with cannabis.

The Utah law has become the subject of considerable controversy among cannabis historians. According to some authorities, the motivation behind this law was somewhat different from that leading to other anticannabis laws in the West (xenophobia). These authorities suggest that a number of Mormon missionaries returning from assignments to Mexico in the mid-1910s brought with them the practice of smoking marijuana, a practice that they had learned in Mexico and that was quickly condemned by the church as opposed to doctrine (as was and is the use of all other kinds of psychoactive substances). In any case, according to this reading of history, the synod of the Mormon church banned the use of marijuana among all church members in August 1915, and two months later, the state legislature passed similar legislation (as was commonly the case with other church prohibitions at the time in the state). The classic statement of this view can be found in Whitebread (1995).

A number of observers have rejected this analysis of the origin of Utah's early drug law. They suggest that religious attitudes had little or nothing to do about its evolution. They argue that the Utah law may actually have been drafted on the model of the earlier California law, and that Utah legislators actually were barely familiar with cannabis when they adopted the law. According to one writer arguing for this view of history:

> There is no hint whatsoever that Utah's law—which, you now see, did not specially target marijuana, and did not even show any particular awareness of marijuana, but merely incorporated the language used by other entities to name marijuana among a whole host of regulated drugs—was spurred by religious concerns. There is no discussion of marijuana, no complaint about its use, no report of arrest for intoxicated behavior other than alcohol or Chinese opium use, no marijuana-related editorials, in Utah's newspapers before the passage of the 1915 law. (Parshell 2012; Parshell is probably the best single source for this interpretation of the origins of the Utah law)

Federal Cannabis Laws

During the first third of the 20th century, then, a movement developed throughout the United States in which the public's perception of cannabis was transformed from a medically useful, commercially valuable, relatively harmless recreational drug into a highly dangerous product on par with cocaine, heroin, and opium. A key figure in that movement was Harry J. Anslinger, the first commissioner of the U.S. Treasury's Federal Bureau of Narcotics (FBN). Anslinger had attended (but not graduated from) Altoona (Pennsylvania) Business College and worked at the Pennsylvania Railroad. Physically ineligible for military service in World War I (he was blind in one eye), Anslinger volunteered instead to work at the War Department. He was later transferred to the State Department because of his fluency in German. After the war, he was transferred again, this time to the Department of the Treasury, where he became interested in problems related to the transport and use of illegal substances such as alcohol (then illegal because of the 18th Amendment), cocaine, and opiates. In 1929, Anslinger was appointed assistant commissioner at the U.S. Bureau of Prohibition (created by the 18th Amendment), a position he held only briefly before being selected as the first commissioner of the newly created Federal Bureau of Narcotics in 1930. Anslinger remained at his post until 1970, five years before his death. Throughout that time, he remained an ardent and aggressive foe of all forms of mind-altering substances, including marijuana.

During this period of time, Anslinger continued to carry on an attack against the production, distribution, and use of cannabis that was strong on invective and weak on scientific accuracy. His broadsides against the use of marijuana carry strong racist tones of the type identified by Bonnie and Whitebread (1970), only focusing more strongly on the supposedly low moral character of African Americans. He also drew special attention to other supposedly corrupt groups of individuals, such as jazz musicians (who were generally also African American), whom "everyone acknowledged" as being of poor moral character (see, for example, Guither 2012; "Harry J. Anslinger Quotes/Quotations" 1912; "Statement of H. J. Anslinger" 2012; for an analysis of the racist basis of many of Anslinger's comment, see especially Moran 2011). An example of the image that Anslinger attempted to portray of marijuana can be found in his testimony before the Ways and Means Committee of the U.S. House of Representatives during its consideration of the 1937 Marihuana Tax Act (which was later adopted). The drug, he said, first produces feelings of "well-being [and] a happy, jovial mood." However, he went on, that euphoria is soon replaced by much less salubrious emotions, including:

a more-or-less delirious state ... during which [users] are temporarily, at least, irresponsible and liable to commit violent crimes ... [and] releases inhibitions of an antisocial nature which dwell within the individual ... Then follow errors of sense, false convictions and the predominance of extravagant ideas where all sense of value seems to disappear.

The deleterious, even vicious, qualities of the drug render it highly dangerous to the mind and body upon which it operates to destroy the will, cause one to lose the power of connected thought, producing imaginary delectable situations and gradually weakening the physical powers. Its use frequently leads to insanity. (quoted in Taxation of Marihuana 1937)

The Marihuana Tax Act of 1937

By the mid-1930s, Anslinger's efforts (and those of his colleagues in the fight against cannabis) had begun to bear fruit. The first concrete accomplishment in that fight was passage in 1937 of the Marihuana Tax Act. (Note that the modern spelling of the substance, marijuana, is of relatively recent origin, with an "h" instead of a "j" being more common historically.) Consideration of the act before the House Ways and Means Committee (presented first as H.R. 6385 and later redesignated as H.R. 6906) began on April 27, 1937, and ran for a total of six days. In his analysis of the hearings on the bill, marijuana historian and then professor of law at the University of Southern California Charles Whitebread has commented on the relatively brief amount of time spent in hearing testimony, "one hour, on each of two mornings," a surprisingly short time for consideration of a major bill (Whitebread 1995). During this period, testimony was received from three groups of individuals, representatives of the U.S. government, including especially Harry Anslinger, but also including the consulting chemist at the Department of the Treasury and the assistant general counsel at Treasury; representatives from the hemp industry, including rope-making, hemp seed oil, and other companies; and representatives from the medical community.

This testimony was almost universally supportive of the bill, especially, of course, from Anslinger and other government officials. Hemp company representatives were also supportive, arguing that they would have no problem obtaining hemp for their products from East Asia (a proposition that proved to be dubious with the start of World War II four years later) and replacements for hemp seed oil. The birdseed industry requested and received an exemption by promising to use only "denatured" seeds, that is, those that were free of THC (Whitebread 1995). The only objection to the pending bill came from Dr. William C. Woodward, a representative of the American Medical Association (AMA), an organization which had also submitted a letter to the committee opposing the bill. Woodward pointed out that there was no scientific evidence suggesting that marijuana is a harmful drug, so there was no reason to ban its manufacture and use.

Woodward's testimony was apparently not what the committee wanted to hear. During one of his appearances before the committee, one member observed: "Doctor, if you can't say something good about what we are trying to do, why don't you go home?" Immediately following that observation, a second member said, "Doctor, if you haven't got something better to say than that, we are sick of hearing you" (quoted in Whitebread 1995). Other testimony had apparently convinced the committee of the validity and necessity of H.R. 6906, and the bill was adopted on October 1, 1937.

The bill that Congress finally passed did not specifically outlaw the production, sale, or consumption of marijuana, but it did impose a complex system of taxes and regulations. Anyone involved in any of these activities had to register with the federal government and pay a tax for each type of activity. For example, anyone who grew or processed a cannabis product had to pay a tax of $24 annually (equivalent to about $360 in current dollars). The tax for sale of a cannabis product to anyone who already held a license was $1 per transaction (about $15 in current dollars), but $100 (about $1,500 in current dollars) to anyone who did not hold such a license ("Marihuana Tax Act of 1937" 2012, Section 2). Federal authorities did not take long to put the Marihuana Tax Act into effect. On October 1, 1937—the day the bill was adopted—they arrested two men in Denver, Colorado, for possession (Moses Baca) and selling (Samuel Caldwell) marijuana. Judge Foster Symes sentenced Baca to 18 months in jail, and Caldwell to four years at hard labor and a $1,000 fine ("The First Pot POW" 2012). Note that some observers dispute this story. See, for example, "Compilation of Publications" 2012.

1951 Boggs Amendment to the Harrison Narcotic Act

In the three decades following the adoption of the Marihuana Tax Act of 1937, Congress struggled to refine and improve U.S. drug laws to deal with two major questions: (1) What is the status of marijuana in comparison with other illegal drugs, such as cocaine and the opiates? and (2) What is the most effective mechanism for reducing the spread of marijuana use among the general population? This struggle led to a number of legislative acts, the next most important of which chronologically was the Boggs Act, an amendment to the Narcotic Drugs Import and Export Act of 1932. The Boggs bill was inspired by an apparent increase in drug use among young people in the United States after the conclusion of World War II. Representative Thomas Hale Boggs, Sr. introduced into the *Congressional Record* reports from local media and authorities documenting this increase. He summarized these reports by saying that "[t]he most shocking part about these figures is the fact that there has been an alarming increase in drug addiction among younger persons. . . . We need only to recall what we have read in the papers in the past week to realize that more and more younger people are falling into the clutches of unscrupulous dope peddlers" (Congressional Record 1951, 8198). Boggs went on to say that the solution to the mushrooming problem of youth drug addiction was the imposition by Congress of more severe penalties for drug use:

> Short sentences do not deter. In districts where we get good sentences the traffic does not flourish. . . . There should be

a minimum sentence for the second offense. The commercialized transaction, the peddler, the smuggler, those who traffic in narcotics, on the second offense if there were a minimum sentence of 5 years without probation or parole, I think it would just about dry up the traffic. (Congressional Record 1951, 8198; for a more complete discussion of this topic, see Bonnie and Whitebread 1970, Chapter 6)

The Boggs Act was adopted by the Congress and became law on November 2, 1951, as 21 U.S.C. 174. The Boggs Act was significant in a number of ways, primarily in the dramatic increase in penalties it provided for drug possession and use. It established a minimum mandatory sentence of two years for simple possession of marijuana, cocaine, or heroin, with a maximum sentence of five years; a minimum of five years and a maximum of 10 years for a second offense; and a minimum of 10 years and a maximum of 15 years for a third offense. In addition, the Boggs Act was significant in that it was the first time that marijuana, cocaine, and opiates had been included together in a single piece of federal legislation.

The Boggs amendment was important not only as a piece of federal legislation, but also because it served as a model that the federal government urged states to use for their own laws. Many states took up the suggestion. Between 1953 and 1956, "mini-Boggs" bills were passed in 26 states. Some of the bills carried penalties significantly more severe than those in the federal bill. The law in Louisiana, for example, provided for a 5- to 99-year sentence without the possibility of parole, probation, or suspension of sentence for sale or possession of any illegal substance (Bonnie and Whitebread 1974, 210). Similarly, Virginia adopted a mini-Boggs law that made possession of marijuana the most severely punished crime in the state. While first-degree murder earned a mandatory 15-year minimum sentence and rape, a mandatory 10-year sentence, possession of marijuana drew a mandatory minimum of 20 years, and sale of the drug, a mandatory minimum of 40 years (Whitebread 1995).

Narcotics Control Act of 1956

One of the signature legislative events of the early 1950s was the appointment of the U.S. Senate Special Committee to Investigate Crime in Interstate Commerce, chaired by Senator Estes Kefauver (D-TN) and widely known, therefore, as the Kefauver Committee. The committee had been formed due to a growing concern in Congress and throughout the United States about the growing threat posed by organized crime. The issue of narcotic drugs became part of the committee's deliberations partly because antidrug activists such as Harry Anslinger attempted to show that drugs were the primary cause of half of all crime in U.S. metropolitan areas and up to a quarter of all crimes nationwide, according to one witness before the committee (King 1972, Chapter 14).

The committee's final report included a total of 22 recommendations for action by the federal government, and seven additional recommendations for state action. Of those recommendations, only one was ever enacted into law: the Boggs amendment of 1951 (discussed previously). Another possibly more important long-term effect of the Kefauver Committee's deliberations was an increasing awareness of the nation's growing drug problem. Interestingly enough, not everyone deemed drugs to be as much of a threat as did Anslinger, Boggs, and a number of other legislators. In the period following the Kefauver hearings, these individuals and the organizations they represented (e.g., the American Bar Association, the American Medical Association, and the U.S. Public Health Service) began to call for a relaxation in the battle against illegal drug use, even calling for the legalization of some types of drug use. This movement produced prodecriminalization articles such as "Make Dope Legal," "Should We Legalize Narcotics?", "We're Bungling the Narcotics Problem . . . How Much of a Menace Is the Drug Menace? . . . The Dope Addict-Criminal or Patient?", "This Problem of Narcotic Addiction: Let's Face It Sensibly," and "Let's Stop This Narcotics Hysteria!" (King 1972, Chapter 14). These articles often called for dealing with drug abuse as a medical, social, or psychological problem rather than as a crime. The Bureau of Narcotics and its allies, as would be expected, fought back vigorously against this view of substance abuse, with its own release of fact sheets, articles, and other publications reiterating the threat that illegal drug use posed to human health and public stability.

This battle came to a head in February 1955, when Senator Price Daniel (D-TX) submitted Senate Resolution 60 calling for the formation of a committee to investigate ways of expanding and improving the nation's laws that dealt with drug abuse. A year later, the Daniel subcommittee submitted its report to the full Senate. That report contained much of the verbiage that had been used when discussing drug abuse over the preceding two decades. It said that drug abuse was spreading with "cancerous rapidity" throughout the nation. It called for more severe penalties for drug abuse and for those who could not be cured of their habit, placement "in a quarantine type of confinement or isolation" (King 1972, Chapter 16). The subcommittee also devoted about half of its final report to disputing the position that drug abuse should be considered as something other than a criminal problem. It concluded that

> To permit a governmental institution to engage in the ghastly traffic in narcotics is to give the Government the authority to render unto its citizens certain death without due process of law. (quoted in King 1972, Chapter 16; for a contemporaneous report on the subcommittee report, see "Investigations: The Problem of Dope" 1956, 196)

Congress was apparently convinced by these arguments, passing the Narcotic Control Act of 1956 without dissent. The act was signed by President Dwight D. Eisenhower on July 18, 1956. The key provisions of the act included even more severe penalties for the sale of and trafficking in illegal substances, with a mandatory minimum sentence of five years and a mandatory maximum of 10 years for all subsequent violations. In addition, judges were prohibited from suspending sentences or providing probation for convicted offenders (Hudon 1956). Finally, some of the more constructive recommendations of the Daniel sub-committee such as developing an educational program to reduce youth drug use and the opening of federal narcotics hospitals to people who were addicted to drugs, did not make it into the final bill, essentially excluding prevention and treatment as possible options for dealing with drug abuse in the United States (King 1972, Chapter 16).

Controlled Substances Act of 1970

Between 1937 and 1969, the prohibition of marijuana distribution and use was enshrined in a cluster of legislation that included the Marihuana Tax Act of 1937, the 1951 Boggs Amendment to the Harrison Narcotic Act, the Narcotics Control Act of 1956, and a hodgepodge of state and local laws. In 1969, that system fell apart when the U.S. Supreme Court ruled that essential elements in the 1937 tax act were unconstitutional. The relevant case, *Leary v. United States*, arose as the result of the 1965 arrest of Dr. Timothy Leary, psychologist, writer, sometime Harvard University faculty member, and vigorous proponent of drug legalization. Leary, his girlfriend, and two children were returning from an extended visit to Mexico when federal agents found a small amount of marijuana in his daughter's clothing. Leary took responsibility for his daughter's having the drug and was charged with possession of an illegal drug, sentenced to 30 days in jail, and fined $30,000. Leary appealed the sentence, and the case worked its way to the highest court in the land, which handed down its decision on May 19, 1969. The case was the first time the U.S. Supreme Court had acted on a case related to the nation's marijuana laws.

In its decision, the Court ruled unanimously that the marijuana tax act was unconstitutional because it exposed an individual to self-incrimination, an act specifically prohibited by the Fifth Amendment of the U.S. Constitution. The justices reasoned that

> the Marihuana Tax Act compelled petitioner to expose himself to a "real and appreciable" risk of self-incrimination ... [It further] required him, in the course of obtaining an order form, to identify himself not only as a transferee of marihuana, but as a transferee who had not registered and paid the occupational tax under §§ 4751-4753. Section 4773 directed that this information be conveyed by the Internal Revenue Service to state and local law enforcement officials on request.
>
> Petitioner had ample reason to fear that transmittal to such officials of the fact that he was a recent, unregistered transferee of marihuana "would surely prove a significant link in a chain of evidence tending to establish his guilt" [footnote omitted] under the state marihuana laws then in effect. (*Leary v. United States* 1969, 16)

The Court then concluded that

> petitioner's invocation of the privilege against self-incrimination under the Fifth Amendment provided a full defense to the charge ...
>
> Since the effect of the Act's terms were such that legal possessors of marihuana were virtually certain to be registrants or exempt from the order form requirement, compliance with the transfer tax provisions would have required petitioner, as one not registered but obliged to obtain an order form, unmistakably to identify himself as a member of a "selective group inherently suspect of criminal activities," and thus those provisions created a "real and appreciable" hazard of incrimination ... (*Leary v. United States* 1969, 7)

For a very brief period of time, then, the United States had no federal policy regarding the use of marijuana. That situation was not, however, to last long. Even before the Supreme Court decision in *Leary v. United States*, politicians were beginning to grumble about the confused state of federal and state laws relating not only to marijuana, but to other dangerous drugs as well. In a special message delivered to Congress on February 7, 1968, for example, President Lyndon Johnson described the nation's approach to drug control as "a crazy quilt of inconsistent approaches and widely disparate criminal sanctions" ("Special Message" 2012). Congress then began working on drug policy legislation in earnest, producing the Comprehensive Drug Abuse Prevention and Control Act of 1970. The act covered virtually every aspect of drug manufacture, distribution, registration, and use in the United States. Arguably its most important part is Title II, the Controlled Substances Act of 1970 (CSA), which for more than four decades has provided the basic legislative framework for U.S. policy regarding illegal drug use ("The Controlled Substances Act of 1970" 2012).

The CSA included provisions that represented significant changes in the nation's policies toward drug use. The first of these changes was the decision to give up on taxation as a primary mechanism of drug policy and to adopt direct penalties and punishment as a way of controlling drug use. In the act, the United States abandoned the principle inherent in the 1937 Marihuana Tax Act that placing a tax on the manufacture, distribution, and use of drugs was an effective means of controlling the use of such products, and adopted the principle that prison and jail sentences and monetary fines *issued directly* for possession or distribution of drugs, instead, were likely to be more effective in reducing (or eliminating) drug use.

In adopting the CSA, Congress also expressed a different view about the severity of punishment appropriate for drug use. Senator Thomas Dodd (D-CT) expressed this view in hearings on the (as it was known at the time) Controlled Dangerous Substances Act of 1969. He observed that

> it had also become apparent that the severity of penalties including the length of sentences does not affect the extent of drug abuse and other drug-related violation. The basic consideration here was that the increasingly longer sentences that had been legislated in the past had not shown the expected overall reduction in drug law violations. The opposite had been true notably in the case of marihuana. Under Federal law and under many State laws marihuana violations carry the same strict penalties that are applicable to hard narcotics, yet marihuana violations have almost doubled in the last 2 years alone. (Controlled Dangerous Substances Act of 1969 2012, 2308)

Reflecting this new view of "the drug problem," the CSA eliminated many of the most severe penalties for drug abuse, including the harsh minimum sentences established by the Boggs amendment. Congress had apparently come to the conclusion that such penalties simply did not work.

The CSA also included provisions for prevention, treatment, and research programs for drug users, a striking change in the previous position that such individuals were dangerous criminals who needed to be punished and/or excluded from society. As an example, the act expanded the availability of methadone treatment for heroin addicts, which dramatically altered the way such individuals were handled in the United States. It also provided for the creation of the Special Action Office for Drug Abuse Prevention, which marked a promising new avenue to research on drug prevention and treatment ("Research and Regulation" 2012).

Additionally, the act reversed a longstanding policy that included cannabis along with cocaine and opiates in drug laws and policies. Instead, Part F of the act established a commission to study in more detail the special problems posed by cannabis use in the United States and to offer recommendations for dealing with those problems. That commission, chaired by Raymond P. Shafer, former governor of Pennsylvania, issued its report, *Marihuana: A Signal of Misunderstanding*, in 1972. The report was an about-face from previous policy toward marijuana, recommending much more lenient penalties for possession of the drug and expanded programs of treatment, prevention, and research. The philosophy that motivated the committee's recommendations was enunciated at one point by Shafer, who said that

we believe that the criminal law is too harsh a tool to apply to personal possession even in the effort to discourage use. It implies an overwhelming indictment of the behavior which we believe is not appropriate. The actual and potential harm of use of the drug is not great enough to justify intrusion by the criminal law into private behavior, a step which our society takes only "with the greatest reluctance." (U.S. Commission on Marihuana and Drug Abuse 1972, Chapter 5)

In some respects, the most significant long-term effect of the CSA was the creation of a system for classifying illegal substances under one of five so-called schedules. This system of so-called controlled substances has dominated U.S. drug policy throughout the more than four decades since the adoption of the CSA. The schedules were (and still are) based on three features of any given substance: (1) its potential for abuse, (2) its value in accepted medical treatment in the United States, and (3) its safety when used under medical supervision. Thus substances placed in schedule I are those that (1) have a high potential for abuse, (2) have no currently accepted use for medical treatments in the United States, and (3) cannot be safely used even under appropriate medical supervision. Drugs traditionally regarded as the most dangerous—cocaine, the opiates, marijuana—are classified under schedule I of the act. Other examples of schedule I drugs today are LSD, mescaline, peyote, and psilocybin. In contrast to schedule I drugs, substances listed in schedule V: (1) have minimal potential for abuse, (2) have accepted medical applications in the United States, and (3) are generally regarded as safe to use under medical supervision (although they may lead to addiction). Examples of schedule V drugs are certain cough medications that contain small amounts of codeine and products used to treat diarrhea that contain small amounts of opium. In the first announcement of scheduled drugs in the *Federal Register* in 1971, 59 substances were listed in schedule I, 21 in schedule II, 22 in schedule III, 11 in schedule IV, and five in schedule V (Title 21: Food and Drugs 1971, 7803–7805). Since that time, about 160 substances have been added to and dropped from one or more of the schedules (Office of Diversion Control 2012).

The Shafer Report

The National Commission on Marihuana and Drug Abuse (the Shafer Commission) took its job seriously. It conducted by far the most comprehensive study of marijuana ever carried out in the United States, holding hearings that produced thousands of pages of testimony from public officials, community leaders, law enforcement officers, academicians, public health experts, and others with experience and expertise in the field of drug abuse. It also commissioned more than 50 studies on all aspects of marijuana use in the United States as well as on the status and effectiveness of existing marijuana laws. It eventually came to the conclusion cited earlier that the possession of marijuana by individuals for their own use should be decriminalized, that is, not penalized by either civil or criminal law ("Nixon Tapes" 2002).

As in other instances before and since, the commission's report did not appear in a politically neutral climate. In fact, even as the committee was conducting its work, President Richard M. Nixon was making clear that he held very different views about the nation's drug problems. He was, in fact, envisioning a "war on drugs" that would be an essential element in his campaign for re-election and a keystone of his second administration. In tapes made while he was in office, for example, Nixon told his chief of staff, H. R ("Bob") Haldeman that he wanted "a drug thing every week" during the re-election campaign ("Nixon Tapes" 2002). At the same time, Nixon was warning Shafer that he could not allow his committee to get out of hand and make recommendations that ran counter to what Congress and the general public wanted to hear. He warned Shafer to avoid adopting the views of "a bunch of muddle-headed psychiatrists" at the U.S. Department of Health, Education, and Welfare who let "their hearts run their brains" ("Nixon Tapes" 2002). Nixon concluded his instructions to Shafer by advising him:

> You see, the thing that is so terribly important here is that it not appear that the Commission's frankly just a bunch of do-gooders, I mean, they say they're a bunch of old men [who] don't understand, that's fine, I wouldn't mind that, but if they get the idea you're just a bunch of do-gooders that are going to come out with a quote "soft on marijuana" report, that'll destroy it, right off the bat. I think there's a need to come out with a report that is totally oblivious to some obvious differences between marijuana and other drugs, other dangerous drugs . . . ("Nixon Tapes" 2002)

Within this setting, it is hardly surprising that the Shafer report went essentially nowhere. True, the report did have some important lasting contributions to make to the nation's effort to deal with drug abuse—it insisted for the first time, for example, to describe alcohol as a dangerous drug—but it had essentially no effect on changing the way the nation viewed marijuana as a "dangerous drug," a perception that has not essentially changed among government officials today. Even as the Shafer committee was conducting its studies, Nixon decided to strengthen the nation's battle against drug abuse by creating a new administrative office to deal with the problem, the Special

Action Office for Drug Abuse Prevention. To lead that office, Nixon appointed a respected physician, Dr. Jerome Jaffe, the first of a series of national drug leaders who were later generally referred to as drug czars.

The Carter Years

The years from 1977 to 1981 provided a brief respite in the war against drugs declared by Richard Nixon. During that period, President Jimmy Carter took a much softer approach to dealing with all psychoactive drugs, calling for reduced penalties for their use and an expanded and improved program of education, treatment, and prevention. With respect to marijuana, he notably observed in a 1977 message to Congress that "[p]enalties against possession of a drug should not be more damaging to an individual than the use of the drug itself" (Carter 2012). As recently as 2011, Carter repeated that message in an op-ed in the *New York Times* (Carter 2011, A35). Dr. Peter Bourne, Carter's drug czar, took a similar view toward marijuana. In a 2000 interview with PBS, Bourne remembered the Carter administration's attitude about marijuana:

We did not view marijuana as a significant health problem—as it was not—even though there were people who wanted to construe it as being a public health problem. Nobody dies from marijuana smoking. (Interview: Peter Bourne 2012)

The Nixon administration's policy toward marijuana use, Bourne observed, was motivate by something other than public health issues.

Smoking marijuana [in the 1960s] became very important as a symbolic gesture against the government. . . . We're really talking more about cultural wars than we are talking about drug wars. (Interview: Peter Bourne 2012)

*Federal Legislation since the Controlled
Substances Act, 1970–2010*

The one-term Carter administration represented only a brief
interlude in the much longer aggressive campaign (the war on
drugs) that lasted from the Nixon administration to (arguably)
the most recent administration of President Barack Obama.
With the election of President Ronald Reagan in 1981, national
policy reverted once again to a militaristic theme in which all of
the nation's resources were marshaled in an effort to reduce or
eliminate the use of illegal drugs in the United States. In one of
his earliest speeches in office, Reagan announced that "we're taking down the surrender flag that has flown over so many drug
efforts; we're running up a battle flag" ("Remarks on Signing
Executive Order 12368" 1982). An indication of the sincerity
with which Reagan attempted to pursue the drug war was the
words and actions of his first drug czar, Carlton Turner. Turner
argued that smoking marijuana was more than just a recreational
activity with young people of the 1980s. It was instead, he told
an interviewer with *Government Executive* magazine in 1982, a
"behavioral pattern" that "sort of tagged along" with an "anti-
military, anti-nuclear power, anti-big business, anti-authority"
attitude that refused to accept civic responsibility (quoted in
Kick 2002, 150; also see Schlosser 1997). When it was discovered
in 1983 that federal agents had illegally sprayed marijuana plants
from the air with toxic paraquat herbicide, Turner appeared on
television to say that anyone who died of ingesting the herbicide
probably got what he or she deserved. Two years later, at a gay
pride parade in Atlanta, Turner also suggested that convicted
drug dealers should receive the death penalty (Herer 2001,
Chapter 15). When Turner said a year later that marijuana caused
homosexuality which, in turn, caused HIV/AIDS, Reagan apparently had heard enough and fired Turner from his position
(Herer 2001, Chapter 15; for a recent expression of Turner's
views on marijuana, see Turner 2012).

The tenor of congressional attitudes toward drugs in general and marijuana in particular in the 1980s was illustrated by passage of the Anti-Drug Abuse Act of 1986. Apparently the primary impetus for that act was an attempt by the Democratic Party to convince the nation that it was "tough on drugs," a position traditionally taken by its opponents in the Republican Party, especially at election time (as it was in 1986). In an attempt to prove that the part *could* be tough on drugs, Democrats pushed through legislation that reinstated minimum penalties for possession of drugs (Sterling 2012). The penalties established for "harder" drugs, like cocaine, heroin, and amphetamines, were relatively large, compared to those established for marijuana. For example, conviction for possession of five grams of crack cocaine, or 500 grams of powder cocaine, or one gram of LSD resulted in a minimum sentence of five years without possibility of parole. Possession of 10 times those quantities called for a minimum sentence of 10 years without possibility of parole. By contrast, a five-year prison sentence without possibility of parole was established for possession of 100 cannabis plants or 100 kilograms of marijuana, and a 10-year sentence for 1,000 plants or 1,000 kilograms of marijuana (Sterling 2012). In addition to re-establishing minimum penalties, the law provided $1.7 billion for drug enforcement efforts, $200 million for drug education programs, and $241 million for drug treatment programs (Public Law 99-570 2012, Section J; also see "Thirty Years of America's Drug Wars" 2012).

By 1986, then, federal laws on possession, cultivation, and distribution had essentially been established. The modern expression of those laws is summarized in Table 2.1.

State Marijuana Laws

As might be expected, marijuana laws vary considerably from state to state. One way to compare these laws is simply to prepare a chart like Table 2.1 for each state and try to decide which states are "most severe" in their laws and which are "less severe."

Table 2.1   Federal Marijuana Laws

Amount	Level	Possession Incarceration	Fine
Any (first offense)	Misdemeanor	1 year	$1,000
Any (second offense)	Misdemeanor	15 days*	$2,500
Any (third offense)	Misdemeanor or felony	90 days to 3 years*	$3,500
Sale or Cultivation			
Less than 50 plants or 50 kilograms (first offense)	Felony	Not more than 5 years	$250,000
50–99 plants or 50–99 kilograms (first offense)	Felony	Nor more than 20 years	$1 million
100–999 plants or 100–999 kilograms (first offense)	Felony	5–40 years	$2 million–$5 million
1,000 or more plants, or 1,000 or more kilograms (first offense)	Felony	10 years–life	$4 million–$10 million
Sale to a minor	Felony	Double penalty	Double penalty
Sale within 1,000 feet of a school	Felony	Double penalty	Double penalty

*Mandatory minimum penalty.

Source: Adapted from "Federal Penalties." NORML. http://norml.org/laws/item/federal-penalties-2?category_id=833. Accessed on January 23, 2012.

An excellent way of making such a comparison can be found on the NORML website, which lists marijuana laws for all 50 states ("Penalties" 2012). As this site indicates, states with the most severe penalties include those that impose a one-year prison term for possession of a relatively small amount of marijuana (typically 20 to 35 grams, or about an ounce or less) and a fine ranging from $1,000 to $5,000. States that fall into this category include Florida, Indiana, Kansas, Maryland, Missouri, Oklahoma, Rhode Island, South Dakota, and Tennessee ("Penalties" 2012). By contrast, a number of states have decriminalized the possession of small amounts of marijuana. Decriminalization typically means that possession of small amounts of marijuana is treated in the same way as a minor traffic offense. There is no prison time or monetary fine assessed, and the offense may not be recorded in a person's legal records. As of 2012, states that have decriminalized the possession of small amounts of marijuana include Alaska (one ounce or less), California (28.5 grams or less), Colorado (two ounces or less), Connecticut (0.5 ounce or less), Maine (usable amount with proof of physician's prescription), Massachusetts (one ounce or less), Minnesota (less than 42.5 grams), Mississippi (30 grams or less), Nebraska (one ounce or less), Nevada (less than one ounce), New York (25 grams or less), North Carolina (0.5 ounce or less), Ohio (less than 100 grams), and Oregon (less than one ounce) ("States that Have Decriminalized" 2012).

Most of the laws in states that have decriminalized the possession of small amounts of marijuana closely follow a model law suggested by the Marijuana Policy Project. That model law specifies that first-time possession of less than an ounce of marijuana by a person over the age of 18 should be considered a civil offense with no jail or prison time and a fine of $100. Individuals under the age of 18 should be assessed the fine (without jail or prison time) only if they do not complete a drug awareness program (Marijuana Policy Project 2012).

Patterns of Marijuana Use in the United States

National Trends

Efforts to obtain valid estimates of the number of boys and girls, men and women who use marijuana in the United States go back to the early 1970s, largely, at first, in response to provisions of the Controlled Substances Act of 1970, which required the collection of such statistics. Research on the prevalence of marijuana use and related topics originated with two studies commissioned in 1971 and 1972 by the National Commission on Marihuana and Drug Abuse (NCMDA). Those studies were then continued by the National Institute on Drug Abuse (NIDA) under the title of the National Household Survey on Drug Abuse (NHSDU), which was later renamed the National Survey on Drug Use and Health (NSDU) and which continues to carry out annual surveys of drug use.

At the outset (and, to some extent, up to the present time), it should be noted that such data were relatively difficult to collect because, of course, marijuana was, and still is, an illegal drug, so an individual might be reluctant to be entirely forthcoming as to her or his use of the substance (see, for example, Gettman 2012). Nonetheless, researchers worked diligently to estimate the number of marijuana users. Such studies commonly divided users into categories, many of which were, of course, demographic: by age, gender, and, sometimes, racial or ethnic background. Also, researchers attempted to distinguish individuals who had tried the drug only once ("one-time users"), who used it occasionally ("within the past year/month/week"), or who used it regularly.

Much of the earliest research focused on the use of marijuana by young people, possibly because of the widespread publicity at the time about the threat posed by drug abuse among teenagers and young adults. In a series of studies commissioned by the NIDA, for example, researchers found in 1974 that 52.8 percent of 18 to 21 year olds and 47.2 percent of 22 to 25 year olds had used marijuana at least once in their lifetime. In 1976, the rates were 50.4 percent and 51.6 percent, and they were 56.8 percent and 60.3 percent in 1977 (Richards 1981, Table 1, 44; the data in this report are taken from unpublished data from the NIDA surveys for 1974, 1976, and 1977). Researchers in 1976 and 1977 further divided marijuana users into finer categories of gender, race, and geographic locations, as shown in Table 2.2.

Finally, researchers asked respondents about the frequency of their marijuana use. The results of that question are summarized in Table 2.3.

Researchers have continued to ask men and women, boys and girls of all ages, races, and ethnic backgrounds over the past four decades about marijuana use. Table 2.4, which is based on these studies, provides a general view of prevalence rates of marijuana use.

The longest continuing study of marijuana use and attitudes toward marijuana use has been the Monitoring the Future

Table 2.2   Classification of Marijuana Users by Gender, Race, and
Geographic Location, 1976 and 1977 (percentage)

Subgroup	1976	1977
Females	43.6	54.4
Males	59.8	64.5
White	53.6	60.1
Nonwhite	46.3	54.4
Large metropolitan	58.1	62.7
Other metropolitan	57.5	63.2
Nonmetropolitan	36.2	47.8

Source: Richards, Louise G, ed. Demographic Trends and Drug Abuse, 1980–1995.
NIDA Research Monograph 35. Washington, DC: Government Printing Office,
May 1981, Table 4, 45.

(MTF) program, known originally as the National High School
Senior Survey, funded by the National Institute on Drug Abuse
and conducted by the Institute for Social Research at the
University of Michigan. The study originally focused on about
16,000 high school seniors in approximately 130 schools. In

Table 2.3   Frequency of Marijuana Use, 1974, 1976, and 1977 (percentage)

Category	Current Use*			Regular Use			Occasional Use		
	1974	1976	1977	1974	1976	1977	1974	1976	1977
18–21 years old	30.3	25.6	30.4	10.8	6.9	13.0	27.0	22.3	23.7
22–25 years old	20.4	25.7	24.2	6.7	6.5	10.7	21.6	27.4	22.6
18–25 years old									
Females	**	19.6	20.8	**	4.4	**	**	20.2	21.3
Males	**	31.4	35.1	**	**	7.0	**	29.2	25.8
White	**	26.3	20.4	**	8.9	12.2	**	26.2	23.7
Nonwhite	**	23.8	24.1	**	6.5	10.5	**	20.2	22.0

*Use within the past month.
**Not asked.

Source: Richards, Louise G, ed. Demographic Trends and Drug Abuse, 1980–1995.
NIDA Research Monograph 35. Washington, DC: Government Printing Office,
May 1981, Tables 10 and 12, 48–49.

Table 2.4   Marijuana Use in the United States, 1990–2010 (nearest 1,000)

Year	Past Month Use	Past Year Use
1990	10,206,000	20,454,000
1991	9,721,000	19,235,000
1992	8,950,000	17,400,000
1993	8,992,000	18,573,000
1994	10,112,000	17,813,000
1995	9,842,000	17,755,000
1996	10,095,000	18,398,000
1997	11,109,000	19,446,000
1998	11,016,000	18,710,000
1999	10,458,000	19,082,000
2000	10,714,000	18,611,000
2001	12,122,000	21,065,000
2002	14,584,000	25,755,000
2003	14,775,000	25,231,000
2004	14,677,000	25,451,000
2005	14,557,000	25,375,000
2006	14,813,000	25,378,000
2007	14,448,000	25,085,000
2008	15,203,000	25,768,000
2009	16,718,000	28,521,000
2010	17,373,000	29,206,000

Source: "National Survey on Drug Use & Health." Office of Applied Statistics. Substance Abuse and Mental Health Services Administration. http://oas.samhsa.gov/nsduh.htm. Accessed on September 29, 2012.

1976, the study was expanded to include populations beyond high school students and to cover a greater variety of topics than drug use. Finally, in 1991, the survey was extended again, this time to include samples of eighth and tenth graders.

As with many marijuana use studies, MTF researchers have traditionally asked students how frequently they use the drug: (1) at any time in their life, (2) during the last year, and (3) during the last 30 days. The long-term trends of "ever" using the drug have ranged from a low of 32.6 percent in 1992 to a high of 60.4 percent in 1979. During the first decade of the 21st century, "ever" use of marijuana has remained within the

40 percent range, with a low of 41.8 percent in 2007 and a high of 49.0 percent in 2001. Throughout the 35-year history of the MTF research, marijuana use among twelfth-grade students has displayed patterns of gradual increase and decrease, with no long-term trends consistently upward or downward ("Long-Term Trends in Lifetime Prevalence" 2012).

Data for "30-day use" of marijuana follow a roughly similar pattern to those for "ever" use reported earlier in this chapter. The lowest rate for 30-day use was reported in 1992, when 1.9 percent of respondents fell into this category, while the highest rate was reported as 10.7 percent in 1978. During the first decade of the 21st century, the rate of 30-day use ranged from a high of 6.1 percent in 2010 to a low of 5.0 percent in 2005 and 2006 (the rate jumped significantly in 2011 to 6.6 percent) ("Long-Term Trends in 30-Day Prevalence" 2012). Patterns of marijuana use by eighth and tenth graders during the first decade of the 21st century for both ever and 30-day use have followed a similar pattern, with a gradual decrease in use from 2000 to about 2007 and an upswing after that time. For example, the highest rate of ever marijuana use among eighth graders during the decade was in 2000 and 2001 (20.3 percent and 20.4 percent, respectively), and the lowest rate was in 2007 and 2008 (14.2 percent and 14.6 percent, respectively), with an increase to 15.7 percent and 17.3 percent in 2009 and 2010, respectively. A similar pattern was reported for 30-day use among eighth graders, with the highest rate in 2000 and 2001 (9.1 percent and 9.2 percent, respectively) and the lowest rate in 2007 and 2008 (5.7 percent and 5.8 percent, respectively), again with an upturn in 2009 and 2010 to 10.6 percent and 11.7 percent ("Trends in Lifetime Prevalence" 2012).

Public Attitudes about Marijuana Use

The Monitoring the Future study, as well as other studies, has been assessing the attitudes of school-age boys and girls as well as adults with regard to their attitudes about the use of marijuana. As might be expected, those attitudes have varied considerably over the past four decades and vary considerably among various age groups, gender, and racial and ethnic groups. An example of those trends can be found in Table 5.6 of Chapter 5 of this book. Those trends suggest that the approval rate for marijuana use among high school students who have used the drug once or twice has ranged from a low of 33.4 percent in 1977 and 1978 to a high of 69.6 percent in 1992. Over most of the first decade of the 21st century, that rate has remained fairly close to 50 percent, with the rate ranging from a low of 49.1 percent in 2001 to a high of 58.6 percent in 2007. As might be expected, trends among those who use marijuana on a regular basis tend to be different, with a much higher approval rating among such individuals. The highest approval rate for marijuana use among regular users reached 91.0 percent in 1990 and the lowest rating was 65.6 percent in 1977. Approval ratings for marijuana use among regular users during the first decade of the 21st century hovered around the 80 percent mark, with a high of 83.3 percent in 2007 and a low of 77.7 percent in 2010 ("Trends in Disapproval of Drug Use" 2012).

Attitudes toward the use of marijuana among adults appear to have followed a somewhat different historical trajectory than those suggested by the MTF survey. The Gallup Poll, for example, has been asking in its public opinion surveys for more than 40 years about attitudes toward the legalization of marijuana in the United States. (Presumably, such questions reflect one's attitudes of approval or disapproval of the drug.) Those surveys suggest that the public has gradually become more accepting toward the legalization of marijuana. When Gallup first asked in 1970 whether the drug should be legalized, only 12 percent of respondents answered in the affirmative, with 84 percent expressing opposition to legalization. Those numbers gradually changed (with only two exceptions, in 1978 and 2002), until, in October 2011, pollsters found for the first time a preponderance of those favoring legalization (50 percent) versus those opposing legalization (46 percent) (Newport 2012). Other public opinion polls have shown similar trends over the years with regard to legalization of marijuana, although none has (as of 2012) yet shown a majority view for legalization ("Illegal Drugs" 2012).

Arrests for Marijuana Use

Perhaps the most relevant and interesting question about trends in the use of marijuana is how they relate to laws that have been passed controlling marijuana use, that is, the number of arrests for possession and/or distribution of marijuana. The presumption of marijuana laws, of course, is that legislation that has been adequately crafted will result in a reduction in the rate of marijuana use. The basic question, then, is whether and to what extent laws such as the Marihuana Tax Act, the Boggs Amendment, the Controlled Substances Act, and similar legislation have affected the rate of marijuana use in the United States. That question has been studied extensively over the past four decades, and abundant data are now available on the subject.

The raw data on the number of marijuana arrests available from a variety of government studies is shown in Table 2.5.

Those data show a slow rise in the number of arrests from 1965 to the mid-1970s, a leveling off of those numbers until about 1990, and then a gradual increase in numbers to the present time ("U.S. Cannabis Arrests" 2012). One might expect to see significant, if not dramatic, changes in these numbers following passage of major marijuana legislation, such as the 1970 CSA or the 1986 Anti-Drug Abuse Act, but such changes are not immediately obvious.

Raw numbers such as those presented in Table 2.5 are not always adequate for drawing conclusions, but more sophisticated analyses (taking into consideration, for example, the *rate* of drug arrests) have produced about the same general conclusions. For example, a study in 2009 by Jon Gettman, former head of NORML, found that "[n]ationally, there is little apparent

Table 2.5 Arrests for Marijuana Possession in the United States, 1965–2009

Year	Number of Arrests
1965	18,815
1966	31,119
1967	61,843
1968	95,870
1969	118,903
1970	188,682
1971	225,828
1972	292,179
1973	420,700
1974	445,000
1975	416,100
1976	441,100
1977	457,600
1978	445,800
1979	391,600
1980	405,600
1981	400,300
1982	455,600
1983	406,900
1984	419,400
1985	451,100
1986	361,800
1987	378,700
1988	391,600
1989	399,000
1990	326,900
1991	287,900
1992	342,300
1993	380,700
1994	481,100
1995	589,000
1996	641,600
1997	695,200
1998	682,900
1999	704,800
2000	734,500
2001	723,600

(*continued*)

Table 2.5   (*continued*)

Year	Number of Arrests
2002	697,100
2003	755,200
2004	771,600
2005	786,500
2006	829,600
2007	872,700
2008	847,863
2009	858,408

Source: These data are collected from a variety of sources, including Marijuana Research: Uniform Crime Reports, Marijuana Arrest Statistics; Drugs and Crime Facts: Drug Law Violations and Enforcement, United States Bureau of Justice Statistics; Marijuana Arrests Drop for First Time Since 2002, Marijuana Policy Project; Paul Armentano, Incarceration Nation: Marijuana Arrests For Year 2009 Near Record High; Drug War Facts: Common Sense for Drug Policy.

relationship between increasing marijuana arrests and rates of use." Gettman also points out that during the period between 2003 and 2007, arrest rates for marijuana possession increased on average 2.93 percent per year, but marijuana use dropped only by 0.21 percent per year, suggesting that arrests were not a "meaningful deterrent" for use (Gettman 2007; Gettman 2012). Gettman also suggests that decriminalization by some states appears to have little or no effect on marijuana use. Colorado and Maine, for example, are both decriminalized states with high rates of marijuana use, but other decriminalized states, such as Mississippi and Nebraska, have low use rates. Gettman also notes that states with the highest arrest rates, such as Missouri and South Dakota, have among the lowest marijuana use rates, but Washington, DC, which also has one of the highest arrest rates in the country, also has among the highest use rates (Gettman 2007; Gettman 2012).

In 1998, the White Office of National Drug Control Policy asked the National Research Council (NRC) of the National Academy of Sciences to review all existing data and research that might be used to develop a national policy on drug abuse. The NRC issued its report three years later, *Informing America's*

Policy on Illegal Drugs: What We Don't Know Keeps Hurting Us.
The main finding of the report was that the nation was spending far too little on drug abuse research, about $1 out of every $107 spent on all types of drug abuse programs, compared to about $70 for drug enforcement programs. That finding led the NRC simply to recommend a broader program of research on drug abuse (Manski, Pepper, and Petrie 2001, 29–36). Another important finding reported by the NRC was the apparent disparity between the severity of laws against drug use compared to their effects. It concluded that, based on available research, "there is little apparent relationship between severity of sanctions prescribed for drug use and prevalence or frequency of use, and that perceived legal risk explains very little in the variance of individual drug use" (Manski, Pepper, and Petrie 2001, 193).

The question of penalties for drug abuse and drug use was revisited in 2004 in a report by the Justice Policy Institute (JPI), a nonprofit think tank whose purpose it is to reduce the use of incarceration to reduce crime. In their report, the authors first noted that the United States in 2004 was spending 300 times as much on the drug war as it had in 1969. Yet, they concluded, "[w]hile spending on drug control has increased, marijuana use remains relatively unchanged," and "[i]ncreasing or decreasing arrest rates had little impact on marijuana use" (Ziedenberg and Colburn 2012, 6, 8). They concluded their report with the observation that

> while the costs of the criminal justice approach to marijuana runs into the billions of dollars, and affects tens of thousands of people through prison and jail (and hundreds of thousands through arrests), there isn't a clear observable benefit in terms of reduced drug use. (18)

Current Controversies about Marijuana Use

Two questions dominate most discussions about marijuana today both in the United States and other parts of the world. The first question is whether the possession and use of marijuana should continue to be criminalized, as it currently is in most parts of the world. For a number of years now, many individuals and organizations have been arguing that there are sound reasons for changing existing policies and allowing the possession and use of small amounts of marijuana without legal penalty. The second question is whether the possession and use of marijuana is decriminalized or not, whether the drug should be permitted to be used for legitimate medical purposes.

Legalization and Decriminalization of Marijuana

In the United States and most other parts of the world today, the possession and use of marijuana (along with its production and distribution) are criminal acts. That means anyone who is found in possession of marijuana can be prosecuted for a misdemeanor or felony crime, conviction for which may result in a jail or prison sentence along with a monetary fine. People who object to this type of policy usually suggest that possession and use of marijuana (but generally not production and distribution of the drug) be either decriminalized or legalized. The terms have different meanings. *Decriminalization* means that the most severe penalties currently assessed for possession of marijuana would be eliminated. A person might still be fined or required to perform some public service, for example, if convicted of possessing the drug, but he or she would not be sentenced to prison. *Legalization* is an even more extreme action, in which all legal penalties of any kind against use of the drug would be eliminated. People who favor legalization often suggest that one or more controls be established over use of the drug, as is the case with other addictive substances such as tobacco and alcohol. They might recommend special labels on marijuana cigarettes, as is the case with tobacco cigarettes; restrictions on all or various types of advertising; age limits for purchasers of marijuana; or restrictions on the amount of marijuana that might be purchased at any one time. Individuals and organizations that argue for decriminalization or legalization often do not specifically say which form of reform they prefer, simply suggesting that current sentencing policies be revised or eliminated.

Arguments in Favor of Decriminalization or Legalization
This section lists the major arguments offered in support of the decriminalization or legalization of marijuana possession. Following this section is a list of arguments used to refute these suggestions and to support existing policies on possession of the drug.

The war on marijuana is far too costly. A number of studies have been conducted on the cost of the war against drug use that was initiated by President Richard M. Nixon in 1969 and perpetuated by all of his successors. Those studies tend to show, in general, that the cost of the war on drugs declared by Nixon increased from its initial value of $65 million in 1969 to $23.44 billion in 2011 ("Drug War Cost Clock" 2012). By one estimate, the comparable cost of fighting the drug war worldwide exceeds $100 billion annually ("Wasting Billions" 2012).

One of the most thorough studies on the cost of the war on marijuana was produced in 2005 by Jeffrey A. Miron, then visiting professor of economics at Harvard University. Miron concluded that legalizing the possession of marijuana would save the U.S. government about $2.4 billion per year and state and local governments a total of $5.3 billion per year. Miron's calculations included all expenses involved in carrying out laws against marijuana, including costs of police, the judiciary, and corrections facilities. In an interesting extension of his study, Miron also analyzed the economic effects of assessing a tax on the purchase of marijuana at the rate used for most other goods or, alternatively, at the usual rates for alcohol and tobacco. He found that under the former arrangement, marijuana taxes would annually generate $2.4 billion and $6.2 billion in revenue, respectively (Miron 2005; this study contains detailed tables for both federal and state costs as well as potential tax returns). In response to Miron's report, more than 500 economists signed a petition to the president, Congress, governors, and state legislators urging a renewed debate on the benefits of legalizing the possession of marijuana ("Budgetary Implications" 2012; for a specific analysis of this issue for the state of California, see GiergiNer 2012). Two other studies contemporaneous with Miron's research also dealt with the problems of financing the war against marijuana. In their 2005 report "Efficacy & Impact: The Criminal Justice Response to Marijuana Policy in the US," Jason Ziedenberg and Jason Colburn pointed out that the cost of the nation's war against drugs had risen by about 307 percent between 1988 and 2003, while the rate of marijuana use had remained essentially the same during that period. (it decreased from about 5,000 per 100,000 individuals to less than 4,000 per 100,000 in the early 2000s but then returned to 5,000 per 100,000 by 2003, for no net change during the period) (Zidenberg and Colburn 2012). Also in 2005, the organization Citizens against Government Waste (CAGW) conducted a study attempting to assess the success (or lack of it) of federal campaigns against marijuana. The CAGW focused in particular on the work of the White House Office of National Drug Control Policy (ONDCP) and found that that office "burns through tax dollars by funding wasteful and unnecessary projects." The CAGW also concluded that "the drug czar created a $2 billion national anti-drug campaign, produced expensive propaganda ads that failed to reduce drug use among America's youth, and in the process, violated federal law" (French 2005). Finally, the CAGW claimed that ONDCP used the nation's $226.5 million High Intensity Drug Trafficking Areas Program (HIDTA) had become a "cash cow for members of Congress to bring home the bacon for their constituents" (French 2005).

The war on marijuana has not been effective.   This point was discussed in some detail earlier in this chapter. The main argument is that the United States has spent more than $1 trillion in four decades in the battle against drugs, the most common of which by far is marijuana, with little or no decrease in use. During the same time, the lives of tens or hundreds of thousands of individuals have been ruined by incarceration for marijuana use. For probably the only time in U.S. history, except for the administration of President Jimmy Carter, an American president has taken a public stand on this position. On a number of occasions, both as a candidate for the presidency, and as president, Barack Obama has suggested that drug use in general and marijuana use in particular should be treated as a public health problem, rather than a crime. In 2010, Obama's director of the ONDCP, Richard Gil Kerlikowske, told reporters that "In the grand scheme, it [the U.S. drug war] has not been successful. Forty years later, the concern about drugs and drug problems is, if anything, magnified, intensified" ("War on Drugs Unsuccessful" 2012). In point of fact, however, Obama's actions did not match his words. He raised spending on drug enforcement efforts by the largest percentage and to the highest amount— about $10 billion in 2010—in American history, representing almost two thirds of his total budget for drug programs ("War on Drugs Unsuccessful" 2012).

The use of marijuana is not associated with serious health problems.   Probably the most contentious issue in the debate over legalization or decriminalization of marijuana is the risk it may or may not pose to an individual's physical, psychological, and social health as well as to the safety of society in general. Opponents of decriminalization and legalization routinely point to a host of negative consequences that may result from marijuana use, often claiming that the use of even small amounts of the drug can have serious results. This argument is in the long tradition of the warnings of drug prohibitionists like Harry Anslinger in the United States and other crusaders around the world, although today's opponents of decriminalization generally present their position in much less propagandistic language and with much more scientific evidence for their case.

By contrast, proponents of decriminalization commonly cite a wide number of scientific studies dating back more than a hundred years indicating that the risks to health and society, although not zero, are acceptably low. In fact, proponents and opponents of decriminalization sometimes cite the same scientific research but draw different conclusions from that research. Some of the most comprehensive health effects reviews are the *Indian Hemp Drugs Commission* report of 1894, the *Panama Canal Zone Mili tary Investigations into Marijuana* (1916–1929), the *La Guardia Report* of 1944, the report of the British Advisory Committee on Drug Dependency (the *Wooton Report*) of 1968, the *Canadian Government's Commission of Inquiry* (the *Le Dain Report*) of 1970, the *National Commission on Marihuana and Drug Abuse* (the *Shafer Report*) of 1973, the National Academy of Sciences' *Analysis of Marijuana Policy* of 1982, and the Academy's *Marijuana and Medicine: Assessing the Science Base* (1999), arguably the most comprehensive review of marijuana-related scientific literature ever produced in the United States. Almost without exception, these reports came to the conclusion that moderate use of marijuana produces no serious, long-term consequences for individuals or for general society. Some of the conclusions reported in 1999 National Academy of Sciences report (Joy, Watson, and Benson 1999), for example, were that:

- "Marijuana is not a completely benign substance. It is a powerful drug with a variety of effects. However, except for the harms associated with smoking, the adverse effects of marijuana use are within the range of effects tolerated for other medications" (5).

- "A distinctive marijuana withdrawal syndrome has been identified, but it is mild and short lived" (6).

- "There is no conclusive evidence that the drug effects of marijuana are causally linked to the subsequent abuse of other illicit drugs" (6).

- "... the short-term immunosuppressive effects are not well established but, if they exist, are not likely great enough to preclude a legitimate medical use" (5).

Proponents of legalization often focus on scientific studies dealing with specific claims made by their opponents about the health effects of marijuana use on the brain, the respiratory system, or other body systems, or on the development of specific diseases, such as cancer. For example, they sometimes point to a study conducted in 2003 by Igor Grant, at the Department of Psychiatry at the University of California–San Diego and his colleagues that showed that long-term use of marijuana apparently has no permanent effect on brain function, a result the researchers found "surprising." In a review of 15 previous studies on the problem, Grant's team found "very small" impairment of memory and learning (Grant et al. 2003). A similar result was reported in a 2005 study of the relationship between marijuana use and cancer. In a retrospective review of 14 earlier studies on this relationship, Donald P. Tashkin at the University of California–Los Angeles (UCLA) Geffen School of Medicine and his colleagues found no association between marijuana use and a variety of types of cancers, a result that they—like Grant—found "surprising." They concluded that although "there is every reason to expect some adverse effect of marijuana use on aerodigestive tract cancers ... results of cohort studies have not revealed an increased risk of tobacco-related cancers among marijuana smokers" (Hashibe et al. 2005, 273). A recent study also found that the relationship between marijuana smoking and pulmonary function is not strong, with marijuana smokers actually having somewhat better lung function than cigarette smokers. The study followed more than 5,000 individuals who smoked marijuana regularly over a period of two decades—the equivalent of up to one joint per day over seven years—and found that they suffered no measurable impairment on a standard lung function test (Fletcher et al. 2012).

When hundreds, if not thousands, of scientific studies on the health effects of marijuana have been conducted over the years, the selection of any specific group of studies may seem somewhat arbitrary. However, these three examples do provide a flavor of the types of results that have been obtained in many research efforts.

The health effects of marijuana are less of a concern than are those of alcohol and tobacco. Proponents of marijuana decriminalization often point to what might appear to be the dramatic difference in the way society views three common psychoactive substances: marijuana, tobacco, and alcohol, the latter of two of which are legal in the United States and most other parts of the world, at least for adults. Studies have shown that the health effects of marijuana use are no greater than, and often are considerably less serious than, those of tobacco and alcohol use. For example, a review of the extant literature on alcohol and marijuana effects on brain function conducted in 2009 by researchers at the San Diego State University/ University of California–San Diego Joint Doctoral Program in Clinical Psychology found that heavy drinking of alcohol by adolescents resulted in significant abnormalities in brain structure, while similar heavy use of marijuana caused "some subtle anomalies too, but generally not the same degree of divergence from demographically similar non-using adolescents" (Squeglia Jacobus and Tapert 2009, 31). In a similar review of studies on the relative effects of smoking tobacco and smoking marijuana over the period of 1988 to 1994, researchers found that tobacco smoking was more detrimental to respiratory health than marijuana smoking on one of nine measures ("shortness of breath"), while marijuana smoking was more detrimental than tobacco smoking in one other measure ("wheezing"), with the two practices having essentially the same effects on seven other measures (Moore et al. 2005, Table 3). How can we justify criminalizing the use of marijuana, some observers ask, when its health effects are no worse than those associated with the use of other legal substances such as tobacco and alcohol?

The war on marijuana results in an imposition on individual liberties. A quite different, but powerful, argument against the war on drugs that the United States has been fighting for half a century is that it has resulted in a broad and intense attack on the personal liberties of American citizens. One of the most eloquent statements of this view has come from Steven Wisotsky, professor of law at Nova Southeastern University, in Ft. Lauderdale, Florida. In a white paper on the drug war for the Cato Institute in 1992, Wisotsky described the ways in which the drug war had empowered law enforcement officials at all levels to insert themselves into the private lives of American citizens, virtually without restriction. He noted that

> the War on Drugs is necessarily a war on the rights of all of us. It could not be otherwise, for it is directed not against inanimate drugs but against people ... all of whom try to keep their actions secret. ... And because nearly anyone may be a drug user or seller of drugs or an aider and abettor of the drug industry, virtually everyone has become a suspect. All must be observed, checked, screened, tested, and admonished—the guilty and innocent alike. (Wisotsky 2012)

In support of his argument, Wisotsky cites a number of both legislators and jurists, including Peter Rodino, former chair of the House Judiciary Committee ("We have been fighting the war on drugs, but now it seems to me the attack is on the Constitution of the United States") and Supreme Court Justice Anton Scalia (the "immolation of privacy and human dignity in symbolic opposition to drug use"). Wisotsky concludes his essay by citing another jurist, Judge William Schwarzer: "It behooves us to think that it may profit us very little to win the war on drugs if in the process we lose our soul" (Wisotsky 2012).

The war on marijuana has increased pressure on prison populations.   An ancillary point raised by Wisotsky in his essay deals with the effect of the war on drugs on the prison population of the United States, a point also made by a number of proponents of marijuana decriminalization. Data on the number and percentage of individuals incarcerated at the federal, state, and local level for possession and/or sale of small amounts of marijuana are difficult to obtain and are often outdated. However, they seem to suggest that, for the most recent year for which data are available (2004), about 12.7 percent of all individuals in state prisons and 12.4 percent in federal prisons have been convicted of marijuana-related crimes. No comparable data are available for local jails, although an estimate of 700,000 has been suggested. Overall, the total cost of housing individuals incarcerated for marijuana-related crimes has been estimated at more than $1 billion annually (although such estimates are difficult to make and subject to dispute) (Mumola and Karberg 2012; Marijuana Prisoners 2012).

Other arguments.   A number of other arguments have been offered for the decriminalization and legalization of marijuana possession and use in small amounts. These arguments include the following:

• The war on drugs has ruined more lives than have drugs themselves.

• Marijuana has been safely used by people all over the world for millennia.

• Legalization of marijuana use could result in a lower price for the drug, thus reducing crimes committed to obtain the money needed to buy the drug.

- Drug dealers would be put out of business if marijuana were available legally.

- The quality of marijuana, its sale and advertising, and other commercial adjuncts to the use of marijuana could be brought under the control of federal and state agencies, such as the U.S. Food and Drug Administration (FDA).

- Individuals arrested for the possession and/or sale of small amounts of marijuana would be less likely to become part of the criminal system, which could ruin their lives and add to federal, state, and local law enforcement costs.

- Smoking marijuana may be, for some people, one of "life's little pleasures" over which the government should have no control.

- Legalizing marijuana may provide a significant benefit to the environment, since the current need to grow the plant surreptitiously does serious damage to the ecosystems in which it is planted.

- In a democracy, adults should be allowed to take part in activities (such as smoking marijuana) that does no demonstrable harm to others.

("Should Marijuana Be Legalized" 2012; Vance 2012; "Pros and Cons" 2012; "Half-Baked Idea" 2011)

Arguments in Opposition to Decriminalization or Legalization
Opposition to the decriminalization and legalization of marijuana has been strong among many individuals and organizations. International, national, state, and local governmental agencies, as well as independent organizations such as Drug Watch International, Drug Free American Foundation, Keep Our Kids Off Drugs, and Save Our Society have marshaled a list of reasons that marijuana and other drugs should not be legalized. In the United States, the White House Office of National Drug Control Policy (ONDCP) and the National Institute on Drug

Abuse (NIDA) have spearheaded the drive to counter arguments made by proponents of drug decriminalization and legalization. Here are some of the arguments these organizations have offered.

Marijuana is harmful to human health in a number of different ways.   One of the most common and strongest arguments made by those opposed to decriminalization of marijuana is precisely the opposite of one of the arguments presented earlier in this chapter. It is that marijuana, far from being safe to use, has many deleterious effects on human health. Opponents of legalization often cite dozens or hundreds of scientific studies indicating that the drug harms the brain, the respiratory system, and other body systems, as well as possibly being carcinogenic. A fact sheet produced by the NIDA, for example, claims that marijuana "intoxication" can cause "distorted perceptions, impaired coordination, difficulty with thinking and problem solving, and problems with learning and memory." Anyone who smokes the drug every day, the NIDA says, "may be functioning at a suboptimal intellectual level all of the time" ("InfoFact: Marijuana" 2012). The same NIDA report also notes that smoking marijuana can have harmful effects on the heart, producing an increased risk of almost five times of heart attack, and on the lungs, with effects that could lead to lung cancer. It also points to research that smoking marijuana can affect a person's daily life, including impairment of several important measures of life achievement such as "physical and mental health, cognitive abilities, social life, and career status" ("InfoFact: Marijuana" 2012).

Statements like these are repeated in different forms by a great variety of government agencies and private organizations at all levels of society. For example, in its drug fact sheet on marijuana, the U.S. Drug Enforcement Administration (DEA) reports that marijuana use may include "sedation, blood shot eyes, increased heart rate, coughing from lung irritation, increased appetite, and decreased blood pressure. . . . bronchitis, emphysema, and bronchial asthma. . . . suppression of the immune system. . . . increase[d] . . . risk of cancer of the head, neck, lungs and respiratory track. ... and headache, shakiness, sweating, stomach pains and nausea, as well as behavioral signs including restlessness, irritability, sleep difficulties and decreased appetite." Some effects on the brain are said to include "apathy, impairment of judgment, memory and concentration, and loss of motivation, ambition and interest in the pursuit of personal goals. ... mental confusion, panic reactions and hallucinations. ... an increased risk of depression; an increased risk and earlier onset of schizophrenia and other psychotic disorders" (DEA 2012; for similar statements on the health effects of marijuana, see "Marijuana Use" 2012; "Marijuana: Health Effects" 2012; "Marijuana Facts" 2012; "Marijuana" 2012).

It should be noted that a number of academic studies have attempted to present a balanced assessment of the health effects of marijuana use. These studies tend to show the potential hazards posed by (usually) smoking marijuana, along with the conditions under which those hazards are most serious, namely, long-term, heavy smoking, especially by individuals who may be predisposed to some physical or mental abnormality. See, as an example of these studies, Hall and Solowicz 1998; Hall and Degenhardt 2009; Kalant 2004.

Marijuana is a "gateway" drug whose use leads to increased risk for using other illegal substances. This argument is a very old and simple one. It simply suggests that people who start out using illegal drugs by smoking marijuana are more likely to then continue drug use, only with even more dangerous substances, such as cocaine and heroin. The American Council for Drug Education on its fact sheet on marijuana, for example, cites a study that claims that adolescents who smoke marijuana are 85 times more likely to go on to use cocaine than are people who do not smoke marijuana, while 60 percent of adolescents who start smoking marijuana before the age of 15 then move on to cocaine ("Basic Facts" 2012). Although this argument is still use by antidecriminalization groups, it has been discredited to some extent by recent research that suggests that one or more third factors may be responsible for the gateway effect (see, for example, Tarter et al. 2006).

Legalization of marijuana could lead to a significant increase in drug-related violent crime. In a paper opposing the California Regulate, Control and Tax Cannabis Act of 2010, which would have legalized the use of small amounts of marijuana, the Heritage Foundation listed objections to the initiative, one of which was that legalizing marijuana would greatly increase the rate of violent crime in the state. The author of the paper noted that "an astonishingly high percentage of criminals are marijuana users," and that, therefore, legalization of the drug would "increase demand for the drug and almost certainly exacerbate drug-related crime, as well as cause a myriad of unintended but predictable consequences." Any income that might be achieved by taxing marijuana sales, the author goes on, would be minuscule compared to the costs of fighting this new wave of crime (Stimson 2012).

Marijuana use cannot be compared to tobacco or alcohol use. The author of the Heritage paper goes on to say that comparisons between the effects of marijuana and tobacco or alcohol are invalid for a number of reasons. For example, he says, marijuana is far more addictive than alcohol, its use usually leads to intoxication (not the case with alcohol), it has no known health benefits (as does alcohol), and it is deleterious to one's health (which alcohol is not) (Stimson 2012). (This comparison between alcohol and marijuana has also been subjected to some dispute. See, for example, Nutt, King, and Phillips 2010.)

The war on marijuana has been effective. Opponents of drug legalization strongly dispute critics' claims that programs designed to reduce marijuana use in the United States have been a failure. They often point to a significant decrease in the marijuana use rate among young people, as expressed, for example, in the annual Monitoring the Future survey. According to that survey, the percentage of high school students who use marijuana at any level of frequency has decreased substantially since the 1990s. A report by the Institute for Behavior and Health (2012), for example, argued that "[t]he decline in illegal drug use is a major public health success and should be recognized as such." Federal and state drug enforcement agencies also tend to point to their increased success in reducing the availability of marijuana and other drugs to potential American consumers. The U.S. Drug Enforcement Administration (DEA), for example, often touts the success of its marijuana eradication program in reducing the supply of that drug to the American public (see, for example, DEA 2012, 48–49).

Only a minuscule number of marijuana users ever receive jail or prison time for using the drug. Proponents of decriminalization often argue that individuals arrested for marijuana possession make a disproportionately large share of federal, state, and local prison and jail inmates. Their opponents disagree and point to statistics that would appear to prove otherwise. In its informational booklet *Speaking Out against Drug Legalization*, for example, the DEA says that only 2.7 percent of inmates in state prisons are there because of marijuana offenses of all kinds, 0.7 percent are there because of possession convictions only, and 0.3 percent are there because of first-time possession convictions. Statistics are similar for federal prisons, according to the DEA, where only 186 people (2.3 percent of all those convicted of drug-related crimes) were sentenced for simple possession, and, of that number, only 63 individuals actually spent time behind bars (DOJ 2012, 61–62).

Other arguments. As with the pro-legalization side of this dispute, other arguments have been presented in opposition to the legalization of marijuana. They include the following:

- Decriminalization or legalization of marijuana will inevitably lead to increased levels of use and addiction.

- The use of illegal drugs, such as marijuana, is generally associated with increased levels of violence and criminal activity.

- Comparisons of U.S. policies with regard to marijuana to those of Europe are misinformed because the history, social structures, and politics of the two regions are very different from each other.

- Even nonusers of marijuana are placed at risk by those who do use the drug. For exampled, nonusers are at risk of being injured or killed in motor vehicle crashes when another driver is "high" on marijuana.

- Legalization of marijuana will increase the likelihood that underage boys and girls may be able to gain access to the drug, as is now the case with alcohol and tobacco.

- The notion that adults should be free to smoke marijuana or not in a democracy is a fallacy because the practice *can* harm others, and some rights do trump other rights.

- The United States and many other countries have radically changed their approach to the use of marijuana, more strongly emphasizing prevention and treatment programs which, however, must be accompanied by continued strong enforcement of drug laws.

(DOJ 2012; "Should Marijuana Be Legalized" 2012; Dalrymple 2012; DuPont 2012; Stimson 2012)

Legalization of Marijuana for Medical Uses

The second major issue related to marijuana in the United States in the early 21st century is its use for a variety of medical purposes. On one side, groups and individuals argue that marijuana is a useful tool in treating a number of medical problems, while, on the other side, groups and individuals say that the scientific evidence for that position is weak or nonexistent.

Arguments in Favor of Legalizing Medical Marijuana

As reported earlier in this book, marijuana has been used in many parts of the world for thousands of years to treat a variety of medical conditions. Many pharmacopoeia, textbooks, and other medical resources have recommended the use of cannabis. Proponents of medical marijuana today often point to this long history, in which some of the finest medical minds in history have recommended using marijuana in medical practice. In addition, however, modern physicians and researchers also point to peer-reviewed scientific studies that appear to support the use of marijuana for the treatment of diseases and disorders such as glaucoma, pain due to a variety of conditions, cancer, HIV/AIDS, multiple sclerosis, epilepsy and other seizure disorders, spasticity disorders, Crohn's disease, and hepatitis C (this list is condensed from Washington State Medical Marijuana FAQ 2012).

The first point that needs to be made at the very beginning of this discussion is that many authorities agree that a large database of research on the medical effects of marijuana is now available, and there is abundant evidence to support almost any claim made in the field, either in favor of or opposed to the use of cannabis for medical purposes. For example, the website ProCon.org has summarized 101 peer-reviewed studies on medical marijuana published between 1990 and 2012, only a very small fraction of all the research reported. The ProCon.org summary lists 39 studies that validate the use of marijuana in the treatment of some medical condition, 31 studies that fail to validate its use, and 31 studies whose results can not be designated as either supporting or not supporting the use of marijuana ("101 Peer-Reviewed Studies" 2012). It seems apparent, then, that the positions taken by individuals and groups vis-a-vis the use of marijuana for medical purposes may be based not only on scientific evidence, but also on other factors such as one's general attitude about the use of marijuana under any circumstances whatsoever.

A few large studies have been conducted to sort through the myriad claims for the medical benefits of marijuana. One of the most important of these studies was conducted by a committee of the U.S. Institute of Medicine (IOM) in 1999, whose report appeared in the form of a book entitled *Marijuana and Medicine: Assessing the Scientific Base* (Joy, Watson, and Benson 1999). The committee claimed to have summarized and analyzed "what is known about the medical use of marijuana." Its report was taken as the gold standard of scientific research on medical marijuana for a decade. Although impossible to summarize briefly, the report suggests overall that compounds present in marijuana, especially THC, have "potential therapeutic value" for "pain relief, control of nausea and vomiting, and appetite stimulation." The committee points out, however, that "smoked marijuana . . . is a crude THC delivery system that also delivers harmful substances" (Joy, Watson, and Benson 1999, 3).

As public interest in the use of cannabis for the treatment of medical conditions increased during the first decade of the 21st century, other research groups repeated and extended studies of the type conducted by the IOM in 1999 (Machado Rocha et al. 2008; Ben Amar 2006; Bagshaw and Hagen 2002; Musty and Rossi 2001). Space does not permit a detailed examination of these studies, but an interesting overview of much of the research was reported in 2009 by researchers at the University of Washington. After reviewing these earlier reviews, the Washington researchers came to the conclusion that "cannabis clinical trials provide empirical evidence supporting the medical efficacy of cannabis" (Aggarwahl et al. 2009, 157).

Among the therapeutic effects that appear to be best documented are the following:

- Cannabinoids may reduce intraocular pressure, thus offering some relief from glaucoma, although the drug's effects are generally no better than those produced by other available medications.

- Smoked marijuana may provide relief from pain resulting from injuries or surgical procedures when other more conventional pain-relieving medications are ineffective.

- Marijuana may help relieve the symptoms of multiple sclerosis such as pain, spasticity, depression, fatigue, and incontinence.

- The use of marijuana may ameliorate some side effects of HIV/AIDS such as anxiety, loss of appetite, and nausea.

- Treatment with marijuana has resulted in slowing the progression of Alzheimer's disease in some experimental animals.

- Marijuana may exhibit antibacterial action that will allow its use in the treatment of certain infections that are resistant to other antibiotics, such as methicillin-resistant *Staphyloccus aureus* (MRSA).

- Some patients with hepatitis C have used marijuana not only to treat the disease itself, but also to ameliorate the side effects of antiviral treatments used with the condition.

(For citations for further information on the therapeutic effects of medical marijuana, see Recent Research on Medical Marijuana 2012.)

A question that often arises with regard to the use of marijuana for medical purposes it how safe it is. Drugs used in the United States must be proved not only to be efficacious, but also safe for users. Studies have been conducted on this issue, none of which appear to show that marijuana is especially risky as a medication beyond the supposed harm it may cause in and of itself (see discussion earlier in this chapter about possible physical risks associated with the use of marijuana). For example, the organization ProCon.org in 2005 requested from the U.S. Food and Drug Administration (FDA) data regarding the relative safety in therapeutic situations of marijuana versus 17 other FDA-approved drugs. Those data showed that between January 1, 1997 and October 14, 2005, no deaths related to the use of marijuana in medical treatments were recorded. During the same period, 10,008 deaths were attributed to the use of the 17 FDA-approved drugs. A second finding of that study was that 9,908 deaths were attributed to the use of FDA-approved drugs for conditions for which marijuana could have been used in its place (thus, presumably, saving some of those 9,908 lives) ("Deaths from Marijuana" 2012).

Arguments in Opposition to Legalizing Medical Marijuana
As might be expected, the primary argument against the use of marijuana for medical purposes is based on the purported harmful effects of the drug itself. Critics of medical marijuana say that the drug is listed as schedule I for a purpose, namely that it is harmful to individuals and has no generally accepted use in the medical community. One would never recommend the use of cocaine, heroin, or methamphetamines for the treatment of medical disorders, they say, so how can one justify the use of an equally dangerous substance, marijuana? For example, the DEA position statement (2012) on medical marijuana says simply that "smoked marijuana has not withstood the rigors of science—it is not medicine, and it is not safe." That view is echoed over and over again by opponents of the therapeutic use of medical marijuana. For example, the ONDCP stated flatly in its 2011 National Drug Control Strategy that "[m]arijuana and other illicit drugs are addictive and unsafe especially for use by young people. The science, though still evolving in terms of long-term consequences, is clear: marijuana use is harmful" ("National Drug Control Strategy" 2012, 21).

In extended debates over the use of marijuana for medical purposes, opponents of the practice tend to offer expert opinion and peer-reviewed research that contradict the claims made by proponents of medical marijuana. They point out, for example, that "no major medical association has come out in favor of smoked marijuana for widespread medical use" ("National Drug Control Strategy" 2012, 25). Such statements are often accompanied by an important caveat, however, namely that certain components of marijuana, cannabis, or their chemical analogs *may* have medical benefit. For example, the major ingredient among more than 400 chemicals present in marijuana is Δ^9-tetrahydrocannabinol (THC), also known chemically as dronabinol. Studies have been conducted showing that dronabinol may have therapeutic effects similar to those of smoked marijuana, but without the potentially harmful side effects that many critics associate with the drug itself. Dronabinol has now been approved for medical use by the FDA under the trade name of Marinol. It is approved for use primarily for the treatment of anorexia in patients who have HIV/AIDS and for the nausea and vomiting experienced by individuals undergoing chemotherapy. In 2006, the FDA approved for limited use a similar chemical analog of THC known as nabilone (Cesamet).

Two other THC analogs now available for use are Canasol and Sativex. Canasol was first developed by two Jamaican doctors and approved for use in that nation in 1987 for treatment of intraocular pressure in late-stage glaucoma. The drug has since been approved in the United Kingdom, the United States, Canada, and other Caribbean nations. Sativex was first approved in Canada in 1995 for the treatment of neuropathic pain related to muscular sclerosis. It was later approved by the FDA, as well as a number of European nations, to treat cancer-related pain.

Current Status of Medical Marijuana in the United States

Marijuana is now permitted for use in at least some therapeutic regimens in a handful of nations around the world, including Austria, Canada, Israel, Italy, and the Netherlands. In the United States, 18 states and the District of Columbia have approved the use of marijuana for medical purposes. Those states are: Alaska, Arizona, California, Colorado, Connecticut (CT added in 2012) Delaware, Hawaii, Maine, Michigan, Montana, Nevada, New Jersey, New Mexico, Oregon, Rhode Island, Vermont, Virginia, and Washington. A fundamental issue related to the legalization of medical marijuana in individual states is that the drug is still listed by the federal government as a schedule I substance, making its use illegal under any circumstances. Various federal officials have attempted to deal with this conflict in one way or another, either by threatening to arrest any healthcare provider who prescribes marijuana for therapeutic purposes, or, on the other hand, largely turning a blind eye to the practice in individual states. At the time of this writing, the administration of President Barack Obama has signaled that it will focus on large-scale distributors of marijuana in its enforcement efforts and limit its interference with smaller marijuana dispensaries that appear to be operating within the limits of state medical marijuana laws (Johnston and Lewis 2009, A20).

References

"101 Peer-Reviewed Studies on Marijuana." ProCon.org. http://medicalmarijuana.procon.org/view.resource.php?resourceID=000884. Accessed on February 12, 2012.

Aggarwahl, Sunil K. et al. 2009. "Medicinal Use of Cannabis in the United States: Historical Perspectives, Current Trends, and Future Directions." *Journal of Opioid Management* 5(3): 153–168.

"Alcohol and Intoxicants in Islam." Muslim Bridge.org. http://www.muslimbridges.org/index.php?option=com_content&view=article&id=1038:-alcohol-and-intoxicants-in-islam&catid=48:contemporary-issues&Itemid=137. Accessed on January 12, 2012.

Bagshaw, Sean M., and Neil A. Hagen. 2002. "Medical Efficacy of Cannabinoids and Marijuana: a Comprehensive Review of the Literature." *Journal of Palliative Care* 18(2): 111–122.

Barnett, Erica A. "Hold the Waffles." http://www.seattleweekly.com/2002-02-06/news/hold-the-waffles/. Accessed on December 26, 2011.

"Basic Facts about Drugs." American Council for Drug Education. http://www.acde.org/common/Marijana.htm. Accessed on February 10, 2012.

Ben Amar, Marine. 2006. "Cannabinoids in Medicine: A Review of Their Therapeutic Potential." *Journal of Ethnopharmacology* 105(1–2): 1–25.

Blanchard, Sean. "How Cannabis Was Criminalized." Independent Drug Monitoring Unit. http://www.idmu.co .uk/historical.htm. Accessed on January 14, 2012.

Bonné, Jon. "For Hemp Foods, A Decisive Moment." Cannabis News. http://cannabisnews.com/news/12/ thread12467.shtml. Accessed on December 26, 2011.

Bonnie, Richard J., and Charles H. Whitebread. 1970. "The Forbidden Fruit and the Tree of Knowledge: An Inquiry into the Legal History of American Marijuana Prohibition." *Virginia Law Review* 56(6): 971–1169. Also available online at http://www.druglibrary.org/schaffer/library/studies/vlr/ vlrtoc.htm (not paginated).

Bonnie, Richard J., and Charles H. Whitebread. 1974. *The Marihuana Conviction*. Charlottesville: University of Virginia Press.

"Budgetary Implications of Marijuana Prohibition in the United States." http://economics.about.com/gi/o.htm?zi=1/ XJ&zTi=1&sdn=economics&cdn=education&tm=36&gps =411_62_1264_564&f=20&su=p284.13.342.ip_&tt=2 &bt=1&bts=1&zu=http%3A//www.prohibitioncosts.org/ endorsers.html. Accessed on February 9, 2012.

"The Cannabis Problem: A Note on the Problem and the History of International Action." UN Office on Drugs and Crime. http://www.unodc.org/unodc/en/data-and-analysis/ bulletin/bulletin_1962-01-01_4_page005.html. Accessed on January 13, 2012.

Carter, Jimmy. "Call off the Global Drug War." *New York Times*. June 17, 2011, A35. Also available online at http:// www.nytimes.com/2011/06/17/opinion/17carter.html.

Carter, Jimmy. "Drug Abuse Message to Congress." http://
www.presidency.ucsb.edu/ws/index.php?pid=7908
#axzz1PSLOq2Hj. Accessed on January 22, 2012.

Christen, Arden G., Ben Z. Swanson, Elbert D. Glover, and
Allen H. Henderson. 1982. "Smokeless Tobacco: The
Folklore and Social History of Snuffing, Sneezing, Dipping,
and Chewing." *Journal of the American Dental Association*
105: 821–829. Also available online at http://legacy.library
.ucsf.edu/tid/rki21b00/pdf;jsessionid=5B96384CF35048
E2F041DEA0934D80A6.tobacco03.

Committee on the Judiciary, U.S. Senate. "Controlled
Dangerous Substances Act of 1969." Senate Report No. 613,
91st Congress, 1st Session. Also available online at http://ftp
.resource.org/gao.gov/91-513/000050F5.pdf.

"Compilation of Publications, Interviews, Criminal Files and
Photographs of Moses Baca & Samuel Caldwell." Uncle
Mike's Library. http://www.unclemikesresearch.com/u-s
-district-court-denver-colorado-imposes-first-federal
-marihuana-law-penalties/. Accessed on January 18, 2012.

"Controlled Dangerous Substances Act of 1969." Report of the
Committee on the Judiciary United States Senate. http://
bulk.resource.org/gao.gov/91-513/000050F5.pdf. Accessed
on October 1, 2012.

"The Controlled Substances Act of 1970." Catholic University
of America. http://counsel.cua.edu/fedlaw/csa1970.cfm.
Accessed on January 20, 2012.

"Controlled Substances Schedule." Office of Diversion
Control. Drug Enforcement Administration. http://www
.deadiversion.usdoj.gov/schedules/. Accessed on January 20,
2012.

Dalrymple, Theodore. "Don't Legalize Drugs." City Journal.
http://www.city-journal.org/html/7_2_a1.html. Accessed on
February 12, 2012.

"Deaths from Marijuana v. 17 FDA-Approved Drugs." ProCon.org. http://medicalmarijuana.procon.org/view .resource.php?resourceID=145. Accessed on February 13, 2012.

"Drug Fact Sheet: Marijuana." U.S. Drug Enforcement Administration. http://www.justice.gov/dea/pubs/abuse/ drug_data_sheets/Marijuana.pdf. Accessed on February 10, 2012.

"Drug War Cost Clock Updated for 2011." Action America. http://actionamerica.org/drugs/wodclock.shtml. Accessed on February 2, 2012.

DuPont, Robert L. "Why We Should Not Legalize Marijuana." http://www.cnbc.com/id/36267223/Why_We_Should _Not_Legalize_Marijuana. Accessed on February 12, 2012.

"The First Pot POW." NORML. http://norml.org/ component/zoo/category/the-first-pot-pow. Accessed on January 18, 2012.

Fletcher, Mark J., et al. 2012. "Association between Marijuana Exposure and Pulmonary Function over 20 Years." *JAMA*. 307(2): 173–181. Also available online at http://jama .jamanetwork.com/article.aspx?articleid=1104848. Accessed on October 3, 2012.

French, Angela. "Up in Smoke: Office of National Drug Control Policy's Wasted Efforts in the War on Drugs," May 11, 2005. http://www.cagw.org/assets/reports/through -the-looking-glass-reports-and-issue-briefs/2005/up_in _smoke.pdf. Accessed on February 2, 2012.

Gettman, John. 2012. "Lost Taxes and Other Costs of Marijuana Laws." http://www.drugscience.org/Archive/ bcr4/2Usage.html. Accessed on January 24, 2012.

Gettman, John. "Marijuana Arrests in the United States (2007): Arrests, Usage, and Related Data." http://www.drugscience .org/Archive/bcr7/Gettman_Marijuana_Arrests_in_the _United_States.pdf. Accessed on January 27, 2012.

Gieringer, Dale. "Benefits of Marijuana Legalization in California." http://www.canorml.org/background/CA _legalization2.html. Accessed on February 9, 2012.

Gieringer, Dale H. 1999. "The Forgotten Origins of Cannabis Prohibition in California." *Contemporary Drug Problems* 26 (2): 237–288. Also available online at http://canorml.org/ background/caloriginsmjproh.pdf, as revised in February 2000, December 2002, March 2005, and June 2006. Accessed on January 17, 2012.

Grant, Igor et al. 2003. "Non-acute (Residual) Neurocognitive Effects of Cannabis Use: A Meta-Analytic Study." *Journal of the International Neuropsychological Society* 9(5): 679–689.

Guither, Pete. "Why Is Marijuana Illegal?" Drug WarRant .com. http://www.drugwarrant.com/articles/why -is-marijuana-illegal/. Accessed on January 17, 2012.

"Half-Baked Idea?: Legalizing Marijuana Will Help the Environment." Scientific American, May 20, 2011. http:// www.scientificamerican.com/article.cfm?id=would-legalizing -pot-be-good-for-environment. Accessed on February 9, 2012.

Hall, Wayne, and Louisa Degenhardt. 2009. "Adverse Health Effects of Non-medical Cannabis Use." *Lancet* 374(9698): 1383–1391.

Hall, Wayne, and Nadia Solowiz. 1998. "Adverse Effects of Cannabis." *Lancet.* 352(9140): 1611–1616.

Hanauer, J. E., and Marmaduke William Pickthall. 2007. *Folk-Lore of the Holy Land: Moslem, Christian and Jewish.* Charleston, SC: BiblioBazaar (reprint of original 1907 edition). Also available online at http://www.sacred -texts.com/asia/flhl/flhl37.htm.

"Harry J. Anslinger Quotes/Quotations." Uncle Mike's Library. http://www.unclemikesresearch.com/harry-j-anslinger-quotesquotations/. Accessed on January 17, 2012.

Hashibe, Mia et al. 2005. "Epidemiologic Review of Marijuana Use and Cancer Risk." *Alcohol* 35(3): 265–275. Also

available online at http://whyprohibition.ca/sites/default/
files/Hashibe%20Cannabis%20Cancer%20Risk%
20Alcohol%202005.pdf.

Herer, Jack. 2011. *The Emperor Wears No Clothes* (11th ed.).
Anaheim, CA: AH HA Publishing. Also available online at
http://www.jackherer.com/thebook/.

"A History of Drug Prohibition and a Prediction for its
Abolition and Replacement." Transform Drug Policy
Foundation. http://www.tdpf.org.uk/Policy_Timeline.htm.
Accessed on January 28, 2012.

Hudon, Edward Gerard. 1956. *Narcotic Control Act of 1956:
Legislative History of Public Law 84-728.* Washington, DC:
U.S. Supreme Court Library.

"Illegal Drugs." PollingReport.com. http://www.pollingreport.
com/drugs.htm. Accessed on January 27, 2012.

"InfoFact: Marijuana." National Institute of Drug Abuse.
http://www.drugabuse.gov/publications/infofacts/
marijuana. Accessed on February 10, 2012.

"Interview: Peter Bourne." PBS Frontline. http://www.pbs.org/
wgbh/pages/frontline/shows/drugs/interviews/bourne.html.
Accessed on January 22, 2012.

"Investigations: The Problem of Dope." *Time*, January 16,
1956. Available online at http://www.time.com/time/
magazine/article/0,9171,861806,00.html.

"Is Marijuana Haram?" Ummah Forum. http://www.ummah
.com/forum/showthread.php?88214-Is-marijuana-Haram/
page5. Accessed on January 12, 2012.

Johnston, David, and Neil A. Lewis. "Obama Administration to
Stop Raids on Medical Marijuana Dispensers." *New York
Times*, March 18, 2009, A20.

Joy, Janet E., Stanley J. Watson, Jr., and John A. Benson, Jr.,
eds. 1999. *Marijuana and Medicine: Assessing the Science Base.*
Washington, DC: National Academy Press.

Kalant, Harold. 2004. "Adverse Effects of Cannabis on Health: An Update of the Literature since 1996." *Progress in Neuropsychopharmacology & Biological Psychiatry* 28(5): 849–863.

Kendell, Robert. 2003. "Cannabis Condemned: The Proscription of Indian Hemp." *Addiction* 98(2): 143–151.

Kick, Russell. 2002. *Everything You Know Is Wrong: The Disinformation Guide to Secrets and Lies*. New York: Disinformation Company.

King, Rufus. 1972. *The Drug Hang Up: America's Fifty-Year Folly*. Springfield, IL: Charles C. Thomas. Also available online at http://www.druglibrary.net/special/king/dhu/dhumenu.htm.

Leary v. United States. 395 U.S. 6 (1969). Text available at http://supreme.justia.com/cases/federal/us/395/6/.

"Long-Term Trends in 30-Day Prevalence of Daily Use of Various Drugs in Grade 12: 2010 Data from In-School Surveys of 8th-, 10th-, and 12th-Grade Students." Monitoring the Future. http://monitoringthefuture.org/data/11data/pr11t18.pdf. Accessed on January 26, 2012.

"Long-Term Trends in Lifetime Prevalence of Use of Various Drugs in Grade 12: 2010 Data from In-School Surveys of 8th-, 10th-, and 12th-Grade Students." Monitoring the Future. http://monitoringthefuture.org/data/11data/pr11t15.pdf. Accessed on January 26, 2012.

Machado Rocha, F. C. et al. 2008. "Therapeutic Use of *Cannabis Sativa* on Chemotherapy-Induced Nausea and Vomiting among Cancer Patients: Systematic Review and Meta-Analysis." *European Journal of Cancer Care* 17(5): 431–443.

Manski, Charles F., John V. Pepper, and Carol V. Petrie, eds.; Committee on Data and Research for Policy on Illegal Drugs, Committee on Law and Justice and Committee on National Statistics, Commission on Behavioral and Social Sciences and

Education, National Research Council. 2001, March 29. *Informing America's Policy on Illegal Drugs: What We Don't Know Keeps Hurting Us.* Washington, DC: National Academy Press.

The Marihuana Tax Act of 1937. Schaffer Library of Drug Policy. http://www.druglibrary.org/schaffer/hemp/taxact/mjtaxact.htm. Accessed on January 18, 2012.

"Marijuana." HealthyHorns.UTexas.edu. http://healthyhorns.utexas.edu/marijuana.html#facts. Accessed on February 10, 2012.

"Marijuana: Health Effects." University Health Services. University of Wisconsin–Madison. http://www.uhs.wisc.edu/health-topics/alcohol-and-drugs/marijuana-health-effects.shtml. Accessed on February 10, 2012.

"Marijuana Facts." Parents. The Anti-Drug. http://www.theantidrug.com/drug-information/marijuana-facts/default.aspx. Accessed on February 10, 2012.

"Marijuana Prisoners." DrugSense. http://drugsense.org/blog/drug-policy/marijuana-prisoners. Accessed on February 9, 2012.

"Marijuana Use and Its Effects." WebMD. http://www.webmd.com/mental-health/marijuana-use-and-its-effects. Accessed on February 10, 2012.

Miron, Jeffrey A. 2005, June. "The Budgetary Implications of Marijuana Prohibition." http://www.prohibitioncosts.org/mironreport.html. Accessed on February 2, 2012.

Moore, Brent A. et al. 2005. "Respiratory Effects of Marijuana and Tobacco Use in a U.S. Sample." *Journal of General Internal Medicine* 20(1): 33–37. Also available online at http://www.ncbi.nlm.nih.gov/pmc/articles/PMC1490047/. Accessed on October 3, 2012.

Moran, Thomas J. 2011. "Just a Little Bit of History Repeating: The California Model of Marijuana Legalization and How it Might Affect Racial and Ethnic Minorities." *Washington and Lee Journal of Civil Rights And Social Justice* 17(2): 557–590.

"MPP Model State Decriminalization Bill." Marijuana Policy
Project. http://www.mpp.org/reports/mpps-model
-decriminalization.html. Accessed on January 23, 2012.

Mumola, Christopher J., and Jennifer C. Karberg. *Drug Use and
Dependence, State and Federal Prisoners: 2004*. Bureau of
Justice Statistics. http://bjs.ojp.usdoj.gov/content/pub/pdf/
dudsfp04.pdf. Accessed on February 9, 2012.

Musty, Richard E., and Rita Rossi. 2001. "Effects of Smoked
Cannabis and Oral Δ^9-Tetrahydrocannabinol on Nausea
and Emesis after Cancer Chemotherapy: A Review of State
Clinical Trials." *Journal of Cannabis Therapeutics* 1(1):
29–56.

"National Drug Control Strategy, 2011." Office of National
Drug Control Policy. http://www.whitehouse.gov/sites/
default/files/ondcp/ndcs2011.pdf. Accessed on February
13, 2012.

Newport, Frank. "Record-High 50% of Americans Favor
Legalizing Marijuana Use." http://www.gallup.com/poll/
150149/Record-High-Americans-Favor-Legalizing
-Marijuana.aspx. Accessed on January 27, 2012.

"Nixon Tapes Show Roots of Marijuana Prohibition:
Misinformation, Culture Wars and Prejudice." CSDP
Research Report, March 2002. http://proxy.baremetal.com/
csdp.org/research/shafernixon.pdf. Accessed on January
21, 2012.

Nutt, David J., Leslie A. King, and Lawrence D. Phillips. 2010.
"Drug Harms in the UK: A Multicriteria Decision Analysis."
Lancet 376(9752): 1558–1565.

Parshell, Ardis E. "The Great Mormon Marijuana Myth."
http://www.keepapitchinin.org/2009/01/09/the-great-
mormon-marijuana-myth/. Accessed on January 17, 2012.

"Penalties." NORML. http://norml.org/laws/penalties.
Accessed on January 23, 2012.

"Perspectives on Drug Policy." Institute for Behavior and Health. http://www.ibhinc.org/drugwar.html. Accessed on February 11, 2012.

Pletcher, Mark J. et al. 2012. "Association Between Marijuana Exposure and Pulmonary Function Over 20 Years." *JAMA* 307(2): 173–181.

"Pros and Cons of Legalizing Marijuana." http://www.umsl .edu/~keelr/4380_ss08_wiki/ba0e099eb51f95fb9dfc0d6 d2f268372.html. Accessed on February 9, 2012.

Public Law 99-570. Available at http://www.glin.gov/view .action?glinID=86926. Accessed on January 23, 2012.

"Recent Research on Medical Marijuana." NORML. http:// norml.org/component/zoo/category/recent-research-on -medical-marijuana. Accessed on February 13, 2012.

"Remarks on Signing Executive Order 12368, Concerning Federal Drug Abuse Policy Functions." June 24, 1982. http://www.reagan.utexas.edu/archives/speeches/1982/ 62482b.htm. Accessed on January 22, 2012.

"Research and Regulation: The Role of the State in the History of Substance Abuse Research." University of Michigan Substance Abuse Research Center. http://sitemaker.umich .edu/substance.abuse.history/pathway_6. Accessed on January 21, 2012.

"Review of the UK's Drugs Classification System: A Public Consultation." Home Office Crime and Drug Strategy Directorate. http://www.drugequality.org/files/Review_of _Drugs_Classification_Consultation_Paper.pdf. Accessed on January 28, 2012.

Richards, Louise G., ed. 1981, May. *Demographic Trends and Drug Abuse: 1980–1995*. NIDA Research Monograph 35. Washington, DC: Government Printing Office. (The 1981 report is embedded in the later Monograph 35 report.)

"Sanitary Code Adjustments." 1914. Topics of the Times. *New York Times*, July 30, 1914, 8. Available online at http://query.nytimes.com/mem/archive-free/pdf?res=9B0 7E1DB1438EF32A25753C3A9619C946596D6CF.

Schlosser, Eric. 1997. "More Reefer Madness." Atlantic Online. http://www.theatlantic.com/past/docs/issues/97apr/reef.htm. Accessed on January 22, 2012.

"The Shanghai Opium Commission." UN Office on Drugs and Crime. http://www.unodc.org/unodc/en/data-and-analysis/bulletin/bulletin_1959-01-01_1_page006.html. Accessed on January 13, 2012.

"Should Marijuana Be Legalized under Any Circumstances?" http://www.balancedpolitics.org/marijuana_legalization.htm. Accessed on February 9, 2012.

"Special Message to the Congress on Crime and Law Enforcement: 'To Insure the Public Safety.'" American Presidency Project. http://www.presidency.ucsb.edu/ws/?pid=29237#axzz1k1QdB1Wg. Accessed on January 20, 2012.

Squeglia, L. M., J. Jacobus, and S. F. Tapert. 2009. "The Influence of Substance Use on Adolescent Brain Development." *Clinical EEG and Neuroscience* 40(1): 31–38.

"Statement of H. J. Anslinger." Schafer Library of Drug Policy. http://www.druglibrary.org/SCHAFFER/hemp/taxact/anslng1.htm. Accessed on January 17, 2012.

"States That Have Decriminalized." NORML. http://norml.org/marijuana/personal/item/states-that-have-decriminalized. Accessed on January 23, 2012.

Sterling, Eric E. "Drug Laws and Snitching: A Primer." http://www.pbs.org/wgbh/pages/frontline/shows/snitch/primer/. Accessed on January 23, 2012.

Stimson, Charles. "Legalizing Marijuana: Why Citizens Should Just Say No." http://www.heritage.org/research/reports/

2010/09/legalizing-marijuana-why-citizens-should-just-say-no. Accessed on February 10, 2012.

Tarter, Ralph E. et al. 2006. "Predictors of Marijuana Use in Adolescents before and after Licit Drug Use: Examination of the Gateway Hypothesis." *American Journal of Psychiatry* 163 (12): 2134–2140.

"Taxation of Marihuana." U.S. House of Representatives, Committee on Ways and Means, Hearings, 4 May 1937. As cited in "The Marihuana Tax Act of 1937." http://www.druglibrary.org/schaffer/hemp/taxact/t10a.htm. Accessed on January 16, 2012.

"Thirty Years of America's Drug Wars." PBS Frontline. http://www.pbs.org/wgbh/pages/frontline/shows/drugs/cron/. Accessed on January 23, 2012.

"Timeline: The Use of Cannabis." BBC News. http://news.bbc.co.uk/2/hi/programmes/panorama/4079668.stm. Accessed on January 28, 2012.

"Title 21: Food and Drugs." 1971. *Rules and Regulations. Federal Register.* 36 (80; April 24): 7776–7826.

Touw, Mia. 1981. "Use of Cannabis in China, India, and Tibet." *Journal of Psychoactive Drugs* 13(1): 23–34.

"Trends in 30-Day Prevalence of Use of Various Drugs in Grades 8, 10, and 12: 2010 Data from In-School Surveys of 8th-, 10th-, and 12th-Grade Students." Monitoring the Future. Accessed on January 26, 2012.

"Trends in Disapproval of Drug Use in Grade 12: 2010 Data from In-School Surveys of 8th-, 10th-, and 12th-Grade Students." Monitoring the Future. http://monitoringthe future.org/data/11data/pr11t11.pdf. Accessed on January 27, 2012.

"Trends in Lifetime Prevalence of Use of Various Drugs in Grades 8, 10, and 12: 2010 Data from In-School Surveys of 8th-, 10th-, and 12th-Grade Students." Monitoring the

Future. http://monitoringthefuture.org/data/11data/pr11t1
.pdf. Accessed on January 26, 2012.

Turner, Carlton E. "The Medical Marijuana Con Job." http://
polymontana.com/?p=2053. Accessed on January 22, 2012.

United Nations Office on Drugs and Crime. Policy Analysis
and Research Branch. 2010. *A Century of International Drug
Control*. Vienna: United Nations Office on Drugs and
Crime.

"U.S. Cannabis Arrests by Year." http://en.wikipedia.org/wiki/
File:U.S._cannabis_arrests_by_year.gif. Accessed on
January 27, 2012.

U. S. Commission on Marihuana and Drug Abuse. 1972.
Marihuana, A Signal of Misunderstanding. The Report of the
National Commission on Marihuana and Drug Abuse. New
York: New American Library. Also available online at http://
druglibrary.net/schaffer/Library/studies/nc/ncmenu.htm.

U.S. Congress. 1951. *Congressional Record*. 97th Congress.
Washington, DC: Government Printing Office.

U.S. Department of Justice. Drug Enforcement
Administration. 2011, January. *The DEA Position on
Marijuana*. http://www.justice.gov/dea/marijuana_position
.pdf. Accessed on February 11, 2012.

U.S. Department of Justice. Drug Enforcement
Administration. *Speaking Out against Drug Legalization*.
http://www.ibhinc.org/pdfs/DEASpeakingOutAgainst
DrugLegalization2010.pdf. Accessed on February 11, 2012.

Vance, Laurence M. "The 40-Year War on Freedom." Future of
Freedom Foundation. http://www.fff.org/comment/
com1106o.asp. Accessed on February 9, 2012.

"War on Drugs Unsuccessful, Drug Czar Says." CBSNews.
http://www.cbsnews.com/stories/2010/05/13/politics/
main6480889.shtml. Accessed on February 3, 2012.

"Washington State Medical Marijuana FAQ." http://www
.hemp.net/692faq.html#4. Accessed on February 12, 2012.

"Wasting Billions on Drug Law Enforcement." Count the
Costs. http://www.countthecosts.org/seven-costs/wasting
-billions-drug-law-enforcement. Accessed on February 2,
2012.

Wayne, Sir Edward et al. 1968. *Cannabis. Report by the Advisory
Committee on Cannabis Dependence*. London: Home Office.
Available online at http://www.legaliseinternational.com/
WoottonReport1969.pdf.

Whitebread, Charles. 1995. "The History of the Non-Medical
Use of Drugs in the United States: A Speech to the California
Judges Association 1995 Annual Conference." http://www
.druglibrary.org/olsen/DPF/whitebread.html#TOC.
Accessed on January 16, 2012.

Wisotsky, Steven. "A Society Of Suspects: The War on Drugs
and Civil Liberties." Cato Institute. http://www.cato.org/
pubs/pas/pa-180.html. Accessed on February 9, 2012.

Wren, Christopher C. "Bird Food Is a Casualty of the War on
Drugs." New York Times. http://www.nytimes.com/1999/
10/03/us/bird-food-is-a-casualty-of-the-war-on-drugs.html.
Accessed on December 26, 2011.

Ziedenberg, Jason, and Jason Colburn. "Efficacy & Impact:
The Criminal Justice Response to Marijuana Policy in the
US." http://www.justicepolicy.org/images/upload/05-08
_REP_EfficacyandImpact_AC-DP.pdf. Accessed on
January 28, 2012.

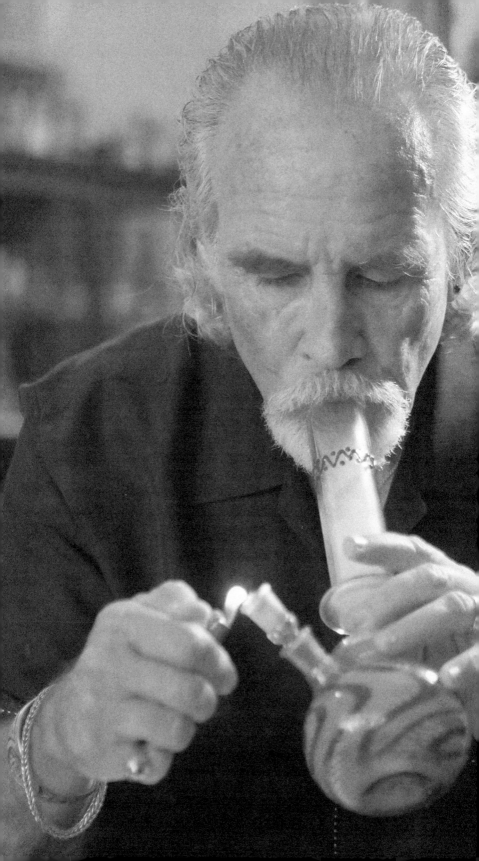

3   Perspectives

The use of marijuana for recreational and medical purposes has been the subject of controversy for centuries. This chapter provides a collection of eight essays defending some of the most common views on these topics. The collection opens with a review by Arthur Livermore, National Director of the American Alliance for Medical Cannabis, on the reasons for using cannabis for medical purposes. Livermore's position is supported in essays by Mary Jane Borden, editor of the online newsletter *Drug War Facts*; Doug McVay, a member of the board of directors of Common Sense for Drug Policy; and Benjamin Radford, science journalist and author of seven books on science-related issues. The collection also includes essays by two of the leading opponents of the legalization of marijuana in the United States, Peter Bensinger, former head of the U.S. Drug Enforcement Administration (DEA), and Robert DuPont, first director of the National Institute on Drug Abuse. Finally, Kevin Sabet, chief of the Drug Policy Institute of University of Florida, outlines some of the specific issues involved in the legalization of marijuana for either medical or recreational purposes.

The use of cannabis has been recommended for a number of medical purposes, including the relief of pain and nausea, stimulation of appetite, decrease in intraocular pressure, and treatment of neurological and muscular disorders. (AP Photo/Reed Saxon)

Medical Marijuana: A Perspective

Arthur Livermore

During the 1970s, when I was a medical student, I was told that marijuana (cannabis) was only a drug of abuse. The knowledge of medical uses of cannabis had been lost. Thirty years earlier, doctors were knowledgeable about medical marijuana, but now it was a forbidden plant. It took me years of research to discover the medical uses of marijuana. My search through the medical school library was not helpful. I found some information in used book stores. There was a copy of a 1921 *Therapeutic Handbook* with medications made with cannabis. When I found Dr. Lester Grinspoon's book, *Marihuana Reconsidered* (Grinspoon 1971), it became clear that marijuana is medicine. How it works was still unknown. Many young people were using it in the '70s and some soldiers returning from Vietnam found that it helped them emotionally. My own experience showed that it is effective in treating bipolar mood disorder.

When I was learning how to control my emotional body, the psychiatric community didn't think that marijuana was helpful. I was given the most powerful prescription medicines available, but my episodic mania continued. I discovered that marijuana helped me avoid these episodes and I began using it instead of the standard medications.

When I discussed using marijuana with my psychiatrist, she was not able to prescribe cannabis because the law said it wasn't medicine. She saw that it was effective treatment for my symptoms and did not object to my use of marijuana.

During the 1980s, marijuana was demonized in the "Just Say No" campaign. At the same time the United States Federal Government was running an Investigational New Drug program that allows patients to use medical marijuana. Robert Randall was the first patient in this program after he sued the Food and Drug Administration (FDA), the Drug Enforcement

Administration (DEA), the National Institute on Drug Abuse (NIDA), the Department of Justice (DOJ), and the Department of Health, Education and Welfare (now HHS). He won this suit in November 1976, based on the medical necessity of marijuana in the treatment of his glaucoma. The FDA's Compassionate IND program was expanded to include AIDS patients during the 1980s. When the George H. W. Bush administration closed the program in 1992, there were thirty patients receiving marijuana from the government. Twenty years later, four of these patients are still receiving marijuana from the federal government.

After the government stopped adding people to the legal medical marijuana list, patients who responded to cannabis therapy worked with political activists to pass medical marijuana laws in the States. In 1996, California passed the first medical marijuana law. As of 2012, seventeen States and the District of Columbia have made marijuana legal for medical use.

In spite of this support for recognizing marijuana as medicine, the DEA has refused to place marijuana in the medical use category. Repeated petitions to remove marijuana from the "no medical use" category have been denied. In 1988, the court reviewed the science of medical marijuana and the Administrative Law Judge, Francis Young, found that "Marijuana, in its natural form, is one of the safest therapeutically active substances known to man. By any measure of rational analysis marijuana can be safely used within a supervised routine of medical care. . . . To conclude otherwise, on this record, would be unreasonable, arbitrary and capricious" (In the Matter of Marihuana Rescheduling Petition 1988). Why does the DEA ignore the evidence that cannabis is a medicine? Quite simply, they are paid to say that all use of marijuana is abuse of marijuana (The DEA Position on Marijuana 2011).

The discovery of delta-9-tetrahydrocannabinol (THC) as the active ingredient in marijuana by Ralph Mechoulam and Yechiel Gaoni (Gaoni and Mechoulam 1964) in 1964 led to the identification of the endocannabinoid receptor system in

1988 (Devane et al. 1988). In 1992, this previously unknown transmitter system was found to be activated by the endogenous neurotransmitter, anandamide (Devane et al. 1992). Exercise stimulates the release of anandamide so the "runner's high" associated with jogging is the result of elevated levels of endocannabinoids. Cannabinoid receptors are found in higher concentrations than any other receptor in the brain. They are in areas associated with pain reduction, coordination of movement, memory, emotions, reward systems, and reproduction (Raichlen et al. 2012; Pertwee 2008; Pizzorno 2012).

Clinical uses of marijuana are not limited to pain reduction, appetite enhancement, and controlling chemotherapy induced vomiting. Cannabis protects nerve cells from damage and is also effective in reducing tumor growth. Multiple sclerosis patients use cannabis to treat peripheral neuropathy. It is effective in the treatment of movement disorders, glaucoma, asthma, bipolar disorder, depression, epilepsy, post-traumatic stress disorder (PTSD), arthritis, Parkinson's disease, Alzheimer's disease, amyotrophic lateral sclerosis, alcohol abuse, insomnia, digestive diseases, gliomas, skin tumors, sleep apnea, and anorexia nervosa (Cannabis and Cannabinoids 2012; Chronic Conditions Treated With Cannabis 2012; Common Medical Uses for Cannabis 2012).

Cannabis is a very safe medicine (In the Matter of Marihuana Rescheduling Petition 1988; Pizzorno 2012). The side-effect of euphoria is one reason patients don't want to use marijuana, but most people like the feeling of well-being that cannabis provides. When patients get too high a dose, they may feel paranoid for a while and then fall asleep. Knowledgeable use of marijuana prevents these negative side-effects.

The irrational marijuana policy of the last 75 years needs to end. Fear of addiction has led to common misconceptions about marijuana. Marijuana laws that are based on the discredited "gateway theory" and "reefer madness" propaganda fail because the truth is hidden. We now know a great deal about brain chemistry. The endocannabinoid system is an important part of our body's regulatory mechanisms.

Marijuana is not going to go away. We must create legal channels for the sale of marijuana so that people can use this valuable medicinal herb without the threat of legal consequences.

References

"Cannabis and Cannabinoids." National Cancer Institute. http://www.cancer.gov/cancertopics/pdq/cam/cannabis/ healthprofessional/page4. Accessed on July 31, 2012.

"Chronic Conditions Treated With Cannabis." http://www .letfreedomgrow.com/cmu/DrTodHMikuriya_list.htm. Accessed on July 31, 2012.

"Common Medical Uses for Cannabis." http://www. letfreedomgrow.com/cmu/. Accessed on July 31, 2012.

"The DEA Position On Marijuana." January 2011. http://www .justice.gov/dea/marijuana_position.pdf. Accessed on July 31, 2012.

Devane, W. A., et al. 1988. "Determination and Characterization of a Cannabinoid Receptor in Rat Brain." *Molecular Pharmacology* 34:605–613.

Gaoni, Y. and R. Mechoulam. 1964. "Isolation, Structure and Partial Synthesis of an Active Constituent of Hashish." *Journal of the American Chemical Society* 86:1646–1647.

Grinspoon, Lester. 1971. *Marihuana Reconsidered.* Cambridge, MA: Harvard University Press.

"In the Matter of Marihuana Rescheduling Petition, Docket 86-22 opinion, Recommended Ruling, Findings of Fact, Conclusions of Law, and Decision of Administrative Law Judge." September 6, 1988. Washington, DC: Drug Enforcement Agency; 1988. Available online at http://www .letfreedomgrow.com/articles/DEA_young.pdf. Accessed on July 31, 2012.

Pertwee, R. G. 2008. "The Diverse CB1 and CB2 Receptor Pharmacology of Three Plant Cannabinoids: Δ9-tetra hydrocannabinol, Cannabidiol and Δ9-tetrahydrocannab ivarin." *British Journal of Pharmacology* 153(2): 199–215.

Pizzorno, Lara. 2012. "New Developments in Cannabinoid-Based Medicine: An Interview with Dr. Raphael Mechoulam." *Longevity Medicine Review*. Available online at http://www.lmreview.com/articles/print/new-developments -in-cannabinoid-based-medicine-an-interview-with-dr -raphael-mechoulam/. Accessed on July 31, 2012.

Raichlen, David A., et al. 2011. "Wired to run: Exercise-induced Endocannabinoid Signaling in Humans and Cursorial Mammals with Implications for the 'Runner's High'." *The Journal of Experimental Biology* 215: 1331–336. Available online at http://jeb.biologists.org/content/215/8/ 1331.abstract. Accessed on July 31, 2012.

Arthur Livermore is National Director of the American Alliance for Medical Cannabis, located in Arch Cape, Oregon.

The Waiting Game

Mary Jane Borden

Like many patients, I make frequent trips to the doctor. There's always that seemingly endless wait. Waiting in the Waiting Room. Waiting in the exam room. Waiting. Waiting. Frankly, I become bored. During one visit after I perused the golf course paintings, thumbed through the magazines left by other patients and scrutinized the proudly displayed diplomas I noticed a consistent presence: the pharmaceutical industry. I decided to write down the names of all the products I saw in the exam room. Mind you, this list doesn't come from the waiting area, nor the hallway, nor lab, nor even the office in its entirety. Merely one little exam room. The list includes analgesics, antibiotics, cardiovascular agents, antianxiety medications, respiratory agents, hormones, vitamin and mineral supplements, and respiratory agents.

Neither does this list represent the universe of drug names I saw in the room. Logos were affixed to posters, calendars, instruments, note pads, pencils and a host of other artifacts. As with stadiums, I expected see signs that read the "Rozerem Room" or the "Cymbalta Closet."

You might ask, why should patients be concerned about this kind of advertising? The *International Herald Tribune* reported one reason. "Spending on consumer drug advertising, meanwhile, has been growing robustly, from $1.1 billion in 1997 to $4.2 billion in 2005, according to a report to Congress by the U.S. Government Accountability Office. In the first nine months of 2006, spending rose 8.4 percent, to $3.29 billion, and was on track to reach $4.5 billion for the year, according to TNS Media Intelligence, an advertising research firm." (Freudenheim 2007).

Further, direct to consumer pharmaceutical advertising all $4.5 billion of it is only one way in which the industry promotes its wares. Drug makers also field expensive sales forces, offer incentives to pharmacies, entertain lavishly at trade shows, dole out free samples and maintain detailed data on physician prescribing and consumer buying habits. In all, the Kaiser Family Foundation estimated that the industry's marketing costs as a percentage of revenue is 34% (Henry J. Kaiser Family Foundation 2001, 13).

With this excessive and costly physician information overload, is it any wonder why, when the doctor finally enters the exam room, cannabis becomes denigrated? After all, advocates of a simple plant can't compete with a multibillion dollar advertising campaign.

Or can we?

What if each of us the next time we visited a physician became reps for our own industry? A wait of any length in a doctor's office will easily identify the pharmaceutical rep: the impeccably dressed individual with a big bag who seems to gain access to the office quicker than any of the waiting patients.

Portraying a rep might not lessen our wait, but getting into the office is what counts. Many doctors, while polite, won't listen all that keenly to the drug reps; they're not patients. But doctors will listen to us.

The recipe? Dress nicely, be polite and carry a packet of professional looking materials about cannabis. Be prepared for rejection; every sales rep should but be persistent. To one office, I carried a copy of Drug War Facts http://www.DrugWarFacts.org, signed it like a rock star and gave it to the physician asking that he keep it in his library of reference materials.

There's an old saying in sales and marketing: repetition = recognition. Perhaps I'm optimistic, but the more we professionally "sell" cannabis to physicians, and as more of us do this on a regular basis, the sooner the medical community will "get it."

But if not, in a mere two years, we'll be reading Sativex on posters, calendars, instruments, note pads, pencils and a host of other artifacts as we wait and wait and wait.

References

Freudenheim, Milt. "Drug Ads Come under Scrutiny." *New York Times*. January 22, 2007. Available online at http://www.nytimes.com/2007/01/22/business/worldbusiness/22iht drug.4291554.html. Accessed on June 14, 2012.

Henry J. Kaiser Family Foundation. *Prescription Drug Trends*. November 2001. http://www.kff.org/rxdrugs/upload/Prescription-Drug-Trends-A-Chartbook-Update-Chartbook.pdf. Accessed on June 14, 2012.

Mary Jane Borden is a writer, artist, activist, and internationally recognized expert in drug policy. Borden serves as editor of Drug War Facts (www.drugwarfacts.org), where she has posted over 1,800 direct quotes facts pertaining to drug policy from more than 1,000 peer-reviewed journals, government reports, and think tank analyses. She is also the Secretary of the Board for the Ohio Medical Cannabis Association (www.omca2012.org) and for DrugSense/MAP (www.mapinc.org).

Common Sense and Marijuana Policy

Douglas McVay

The question has been asked at least since the Nixon administration: Should marijuana be legalized for adult social use in the United States? Perhaps by examining the facts we can at last be guided toward an answer.

If the basic purpose of cannabis prohibition is to prevent cannabis use, then prohibition has without question failed. In 1937, when the Marihuana Tax Act was passed, the market for social-use cannabis was small and limited. Today, cannabis is a multibillion dollar industry and is used by millions of people every day. Many major American politicians and other leaders have used cannabis in the past. They were fortunate to have avoided an arrest, that could have destroyed their future careers—though looking at the numbers perhaps that's not surprising.

According to the Federal Bureau of Investigation (FBI), there have been more than 750,000 arrests for various marijuana offenses annually each year since 2003. More than 650,000 of those arrests each year were for possession. That's quite a few arrests when compared with the total number of property crime arrests (over 1.6 million per year for most of that period), or violent crime arrests in the U.S. (more than 580,000 per year for most of that period). Yet according to the federal government, in 2010 an estimated 22.6 million Americans were so-called current users of marijuana, of whom at least 4.6 million used cannabis at least 300 days or more days during the year. (Uniform Crime Reports, 2001–2011; And those estimates are based on the number of respondents who are willing to confess to illegal activities on a government survey.)

Just because a law is broken with impunity, including by the nation's leaders, is that sufficient reason to change it?

Policies and laws don't exist in a vacuum. A basic level of acceptable risk regarding what substances are legally available for social use by adults has been established de facto, if not de jure. For example, alcohol is available for a price to anyone over a certain age, and is used for its drug-like effects as well as socially. How does cannabis compare with alcohol? The United Kingdom's Advisory Council on the Misuse of Drugs performed an objective review of the health data regarding alcohol, cannabis, and other drugs. Ruth Weissenborn and David Nutt wrote about the ACMD's conclusions in the *Journal of Psychopharmacology* in 2011, noting that "Alcohol was confirmed as the most harmful drug to others and the most harmful drug overall. A direct comparison of alcohol and cannabis showed that alcohol was considered to be more than twice as harmful as cannabis to users, and five times as harmful as cannabis to others." They noted further that "As there are few areas of harm that each drug can produce where cannabis scores more highly than alcohol, we suggest that even if there were no legal impediment to cannabis use it would be unlikely to be more harmful than alcohol" (Weissenborn and Nutt 2012).

A contradiction between policy and science exists. What to do to resolve it? One approach is to regulate alcohol at least as tightly as cannabis—in other words, reimpose prohibition of alcohol. There are several reasons why the United States won't impose alcohol prohibition once again:

Economic—Alcohol is a big industry with millions of users in the U.S. alone. Keeping alcohol legal saves jobs—which must provide considerable comfort to the families of the thousands who die each year because of alcohol.

Social/Individual—The tactics needed to successfully prohibit alcohol might not be tolerated in a free society. The effect of criminalizing a large segment of the population is beyond measure, not to mention the power which could be gifted to criminal organizations. While some indicators of alcohol abuse such as cirrhosis might decline, it's also possible that some behavioral problems arising from alcohol use could increase as a result of the new alcohol prohibition, raising the human cost.

The other option to make controlled substance policy more fair and balanced is to remove the federal prohibition on cannabis. States could be given the option of choosing whether to create their own regulatory systems for cannabis, to legalize only personal use cultivation and possession by adults, or to continue prohibiting cannabis criminally.

The new system for regulating cannabis should be informed by the experience of American society with alcohol. For example: Communities should be allowed to opt whether to allow cannabis sale or to remain "dry," much as is done with alcohol. Other discouraging mechanisms which should be discussed and implemented from the outset include age limits, with hefty penalties for those who would give or sell to minors; reasonable restrictions on driving under the influence of cannabis; bans on use in public or in buildings; restrictions on places when and where cannabis can be purchased (possibly even a state-operated system with no promotions or advertising allowed and very plain packaging), with tighter restrictions on availability in the case of higher-potency cannabis; school-based and community programs to discourage alcohol abuse and prevent initiation of use; and honest public service ads promoting healthy life-styles.

It is appropriate to revisit drug policies from time to time as science develops and sociocultural biases recede, or at least evolve. It is also appropriate to compare cannabis with these other, legal drugs to see whether it criminalization is the most appropriate approach. The facts point away from the prohibition model where cannabis is concerned. By applying the lessons of history, the U.S. may be able to avoid increases in cannabis use and especially in problem use after legalization. After 75 years of failure the laws must finally be changed.

References

"Uniform Crime Reports 2001–2011." Federal Bureau of Investiation. http://www.fbi.gov/. Accessed on June 14, 2012.

Weissenborn, Ruth, and David J. Nutt. "Popular Intoxicants: What Lessons Can Be Learned from the Last 40 Years of Alcohol and Cannabis Regulation?" *Journal of*

Psychopharmacology. Published online on September 17, 2011. DOI: 10.1177/0269881111414751. Accessed on June 14, 2012.

Douglas McVay is a writer/editor, researcher, policy analyst, and longtime advocate for progressive social justice reform. He serves on the board of directors of Common Sense for Drug Policy and on the advisory board of Students for Sensible Drug Policy.

A Case for Marijuana Legalization

Benjamin Radford

In the interest of full disclosure I should be up front about my biases regarding marijuana legalization. Much of what is written on the subject tends to be aimed at achieving a particular political or social goal: either legalizing, or maintaining the criminalization of medicinal and recreational use of the *Cannabis sativa* or *Cannabis indica* plant.

I am not necessarily a proponent of legalizing drugs generally nor marijuana specifically; I have no axe to grind either way. I don't smoke marijuana for several reasons including the fact that smoking itself—whether tobacco, marijuana, or rolled Lipton tea bags (something I toked once as a curious sixth-grader)—is unhealthy and bad for my lungs. I hope to live to a ripe old age, and while something or other will do me in eventually, I'd rather it not be something largely preventable like lung cancer. Make Death work for it, I say.

Some people love Mary Jane with a passion I find hard to fathom; if all the Cannabis plants in the world wilted in the hot sun and disappeared forever it wouldn't matter to me at all (my main concern would be the resulting loss of biodiversity). I'm not going to wade into the contentious debate about whether marijuana is a gateway drug to cocaine, methamphetamines, heroin and the like. I've read that the marijuana on the streets today is much more potent than it was in the 1960s and 1970s; assuming that's true I'm not sure what its significance is, since we are not seeing a resulting epidemic of marijuana overdoses. There are plenty of arguments and counter-arguments on the issue, and many of them are addressed elsewhere in this book. I do, however, have an interest—as a public citizen and a taxpayer—in making sound national policy decisions. My objection to the criminalization of marijuana has little to do with the drug itself and everything to do with the cost to Americans of keeping the drug illegal. Criminalizing marijuana requires law enforcement to pursue and arrest users, dealers, and suppliers. The criminalization of, and penalties for, marijuana use—created by lawmakers, imposed by judges, and enforced by jail and prison officials—are not cheap. Arresting, prosecuting, and incarcerating people convicted of marijuana offenses cost taxpayer dollars that are badly needed elsewhere.

The decades-long war on drugs is widely recognized a spectacular, costly failure (Becker 2012), with a 2011 report from The Global Commission on Drug Policy concluding that "The global war on drugs has failed, with devastating consequences for individuals and societies around the world" (Reuters 2011). Overall levels of drug use have not declined despite billions of dollars spent on law enforcement and incarceration. Of course this in itself is not a logical reason to decriminalize all drugs, any more than the fact that murders continue to be committed suggests we should legalize homicide. However there is a clear public interest in controlling and outlawing drugs that cause significant social harm, and the evidence suggests that marijuana is not such a drug.

Marijuana has been used for millennia and is here to stay, legal or not. The cost of incarcerating prisoners in the United States varies significantly by state and prison, but according to a 2012 VERA Institute of Justice report the price of prisons to taxpayers is $39 billion each year. The total cost to taxpayers for imprisoning each inmate averages $31,307, ranging from $14,603 in Kentucky to $60,076 in New York. According to the report, "In the current fiscal climate, states are increasingly forced to do more with less and make difficult decisions about competing priorities. Policy makers must understand the full fiscal implications of their policy choices, particularly those related to the criminal justice system, whose costs make up a significant part of every state budget. A growing body of research suggests-and government officials acknowledge-that beyond a certain point, further increases in incarceration have significantly diminishing returns as a means of making communities safer. This means that for many systems, putting more lower-risk offenders in prison is yielding increasingly smaller improvements in public safety and may cost more to taxpayers than the value of the crime it prevents" (Henrichson and Delaney 2012).

We as a society can either continue to spend taxpayer dollars on the prosecution and incarceration of casual marijuana users and growers, or we can choose to tax it as we do cigarettes and alcohol. We as a country have finite resources, especially in this era of economic tumult. The $31,307 that taxpayers spend each year on incarcerating marijuana users could be better spent on education and social services.

Legalizing marijuana will not, of course, completely remedy the economic drain on society. The abuse of both illegal and legal drugs will continue. But unlike harder drugs such as cocaine and heroin, marijuana has the distinction of being both a legal and an illegal drug, depending on the circumstance and jurisdiction. Over the past several years medical marijuana has become increasingly accepted and prescribed for pain relief; as of 2012 seventeen states and the District of Columbia had legal dispensaries (Graves 2012).

This raises other questions about the wisdom of continued marijuana criminalization: How much are we willing to spend allowing those with a prescription to use the drug, while prosecuting and imprisoning others for doing exactly the same thing? Society is rightfully willing to spend money locking up rapists, robbers, and murderers, but how fearful should we be of marijuana users?

References

Becker, Alex. "Chris Christie Calls War on Drugs 'A Failure.' " Huffington Post, July 9, 2012. http://www.huffingtonpost. com/2012/07/09/chris-christie-drugs-war-on-drugs_n _1659687.html. Accessed on August 6, 2012.

Graves, Lucia. "Medical Marijuana States Add Number 17, Connecticut." Huffington Post, http://www.huffingtonpost. com/2012/06/01/medical-marijuana-connecticut-17th -state_n_1563206.html. Accessed on July 12, 2012.

Henrichson, Christian, and Ruth Delaney. "The Price of Prisons: What Incarceration Costs Taxpayers. New York" The VERA Institute of Justice. http://www.vera.org/? q=pubs/price-prisons. Accessed on July 12, 2012.

Reuters. "Global War on Drugs a Failure, High-level Panel Says." June 2, 2011. http://www.reuters.com/article/2011/ 06/02/us-drugs-commission-idUSTRE7511WG20110602. Accessed on August 6, 2012.

Benjamin Radford is author of seven books, including Media Myth-makers: How Journalists, Activists, and Advertisers Mislead Us *(2003, Prometheus Books) and* The Martians Have Landed: A History of Media Panics and Hoaxes *(with Robert Bartholomew, 2012, MacFarland). The views expressed are solely the author's and do not represent the opinions or positions of any organizations.*

An Effective Public Health Approach to Reduce Marijuana Use

Robert L. DuPont, MD

The contentious debate about marijuana will continue to make headlines in the United States because of significant funding for campaigns to legalize and/or decriminalize the use, sale, and production of this widely abused drug for personal and for "medical" purposes. I offer my opinions based on over 40 years of work within addiction treatment, the criminal justice system, and in research. A better marijuana policy can be achieved. Legalizing or decriminalizing marijuana is not part of that better marijuana policy.

Some suggest that because marijuana is widely used, marijuana use and the problems caused by it should be treated as health problems only and thus be removed from the criminal justice system altogether. According to this view, the answer to handling marijuana is to decriminalize and/or legalize it ("tax and regulate").

The rates of marijuana use are not static. They have changed dramatically over relatively short periods of time. Marijuana use among 12th graders reached its peak in 1978 when 37.1% used marijuana in the past 30 days. This figure reached its low in 1992 at 11.9%. This dramatic drop in marijuana use reflected an increase in perceived risk of harm from marijuana use and a rise in social disapproval of marijuana use. Since that time, marijuana use has increased to the point that 22.6% of high school seniors were past month marijuana users in 2011 (Johnston et al. 2012). The recent steady increase in rates of use is seen for adults as well (Substance Abuse and Mental Health Services Administration 2011). This recent rise in marijuana use is the result of the pro marijuana campaigns, which portray marijuana use as harmless, and of more permissive state laws regarding marijuana, especially the legalization of "medical" marijuana. The rising levels of marijuana use are destructive to the public health. Strong action is needed to turn them around as was done in the decade after 1978. The public health requires that the dangers of marijuana use be emphasized and the social acceptance of marijuana use be sharply reduced.

The National Institute on Drug Abuse (NIDA) has demonstrated that marijuana use is a health threat, particularly to youth. Marijuana policy must focus on youth because almost all drug use begins in the teenage years and because the teen brain is not fully developed making this age especially vulnerable (National Institute on Drug Abuse 2010). Marijuana policy must commit to mobilizing parents, schools, health care and others concerned with the health and well being of youth to help them grow up drug free. This effort must set the drug free goal of youth not using alcohol and tobacco which are also illegal for youth (until ages 21 and 18 respectively).

A sound public health policy limits the harm caused by drug use, including marijuana use. The best way to do that is to dramatically reduce drug use. Both marijuana decriminalization and legalization increase marijuana use. They thus fail the most fundamental medical dictum, "first do no harm." Keeping marijuana illegal is an important public health strategy that reinforces all prevention messages. The criminal justice system is a strong force not only for prevention but also for intervention to stop marijuana use.

Few people are incarcerated for marijuana use now, but many are arrested each year. I encourage the adoption of community supervision of individuals arrested for marijuana use with careful monitoring to ensure that they do not use marijuana or other illegal drugs for substantial periods of time. I am convinced that brief incarceration is appropriate primarily for offenders who fail at community supervision. This type of monitoring has been successfully implemented in Drug Courts (Marlowe 2010) and by innovative probation programs including HOPE Probation (Hawken and Kleiman 2009) and South Dakota's 24/7 Sobriety. These programs produce excellent outcomes. They reduce drug and alcohol use, they reduce criminal recidivism, and they reduce incarceration.

A better policy to deal with marijuana and other drugs has been widely and wrongly presented as a choice between "treatment or incarceration." This is a dangerously false choice. The systems of health care and criminal justice do not compete when it comes to drugs. A better drug policy is achieved when criminal justice and health care work together to achieve outcomes that neither can accomplish alone. (DuPont and Humphreys 2011) The public health is best served by keeping marijuana use, production, and sale illegal.

References

DuPont, R. L., and K. Humphreys. 2011. "A New Paradigm for Long-term Recovery." *Substance Abuse* 32(1): 1–6.

Hawken, A. and M. Kleiman, M. *Managing Drug Involved Probationers With Swift and Certain Sanctions: Evaluating Hawaii's HOPE.* Washington, DC: National Institute of Justice, Office of Justice Programs, U.S. Department of Justice, 2009.

Johnston, L. D., et al. 2012. *Monitoring the Future National Survey Results on Drug Use, 1975–2011: Volume I, Secondary School Students.* Ann Arbor: Institute for Social Research, University of Michigan.

Marlowe, D. B. 2010, December. "Need to Know: Research Update on Adult Drug Courts." Alexandria, VA: National Association of Drug Court Professionals. http://www.nadcp .org/sites/default/files/nadcp/Research%20Update%20on% 20Adult%20Drug%20Courts%20%20NADCP_1.pdf. Accessed on July 26, 2012.

National Institute on Drug Abuse. "Marijuana Abuse." Research Report Series, NIH Pub. Number: 10-3859. Bethesda, MD: U.S. Department of Health and Human Services, National Institutes of Health, National Institute on Drug Abuse, 2010. http://www.drugabuse.gov/publications/ research-reports/marijuana-abuse. Accessed on July 26, 2012.

Office of the Attorney General. "24/7 Sobriety Program: 24/7 Statistics," 2010. http://apps.sd.gov/atg/dui247/247stats .htm; Office of the Attorney General. "24/7 Sobriety Program," 2012. http://apps.sd.gov/atg/dui247/247ppt.pdf. Accessed on July 26, 2012.

Substance Abuse and Mental Health Services Administration. "Results from the 2010 National Survey on Drug Use and Health: Summary of National Findings, NSDUH Series H-41, HHS Publication No. (SMA) 114658." Rockville, MD: Substance Abuse and Mental Health Services Administration, 2011. http://oas.samhsa.gov/NSDUH/2k10NSDUH/2k10Results.htm. Accessed on July 26, 2012.

Robert L. DuPont, MD, is President of the Institute for Behavior and Health, Inc., a nonprofit organization that works to identify and promote effective new strategies to reduce illegal drug use, and Clinical Professor of Psychiatry at Georgetown Medical School. He is also Executive Vice President and Cofounder of Bensinger, DuPont & Associates (BDA), a professional services company that provides employee assistance programs and drug testing services as well as consultation on prescription drug abuse. He was the first Director of the National Institute on Drug Abuse and served as the second White House Drug Chief.

Marijuana Is Not Safe and Is Not Medicine

Peter Bensinger

Suggestions and legislative proposals continue to emerge on what to do about marijuana use in the United States. Proposed options range from full marijuana legalization, to providing marijuana as a "medicine," to making penalties for marijuana use and/or possession a noncriminal offense payable with a fine like a traffic ticket. These are all bad ideas from a health care standpoint, from a revenue perspective, and from a safety, productivity and crime prevention point of view.

Legalizing marijuana reminds me of the efforts in Britain in the early 1970s to make heroin available to heroin users. Those who registered to use heroin went to chemist shops (drugstores) and received their dosages at purity levels that were well within lower non-lethal limits. The anticipated results of this policy were to limit the negative effects of heroin use (e.g., overdose), to reduce heroin use, and to limit law enforcement needs. In reality, the heroin addicts purchased the more powerful and more lethal variety of heroin still sold on the streets. Rather than reducing its narcotics force, Scotland Yard doubled the number of investigators because illegal heroin imports tripled. Using this example, we must ask, if marijuana were legalized, at what purity would it be sanctioned—at 3% THC, the typical potency of marijuana in the 1970s, at 5–6%, typical today, or 11–12%, found in the "sensimillia" high potency marijuana? What age group could be buyers, 21 and older? The big market today is between the ages of 15 and 25 (Results from the 2008 National Survey on Drug Use and Health: National Findings 2009, 1–2).

Marijuana has 468 different chemicals and 40% more cancer causing agents and four times the tar of tobacco cigarettes (Health, Education, Safety Experts Join White House Drug Czar to Educate Parents about Risks of Youth Marijuana Use 2012). If marijuana is made more available, users will compromise their lungs and incur higher rates of cancer and emphysema. Any taxes collected from marijuana cigarettes will pale in comparison to the social costs of the health and safety consequences of wider use and increased dependence. State and federal taxes on tobacco cigarettes bring in $1.25–$1.85 per pack but the social costs of smoking tobacco cigarettes exceed $7.00 per pack (Speaking Out against Drug Legislation 2012).

In addition to enabling marijuana users to further compromise their health, permitting marijuana users to smoke with no criminal sanction or serious disincentive would pose major problems on our highways and in our workplaces. A recent epidemiological review showed that marijuana use significantly increases the risk of motor vehicle crash (Li et al. 2011). One of the major deterrents to using marijuana and other illegal drugs over the last 30 years has been the adoption by employers, the military and government agencies of fitness for duty as a condition of employment. What would happen to workplace safety and productivity if marijuana were legal and/or its use acceptable or permitted for medical reasons?

In California, a state with a long history of "medical" marijuana, less than 10% of individuals with marijuana cards have cancer, AIDS, glaucoma or muscular dystrophy, the most serious and most common conditions for which "medical" marijuana is promised to help through these laws ("Medical Marijuana" 2012). Over 500,000 Californians have "medical" marijuana cards, most of them aged between 18–35 and almost all of them free of serious medical conditions. The professional associations representing those identified by legislators as needing smoked marijuana are all opposed to "medical" marijuana. After my appointment as Administrator of the U.S. Drug Enforcement Administration (DEA) by President Ford in 1976, I received repeated requests to authorize marijuana for individuals claiming to need it for personal use and well being. I asked what the view of the Food and Drug Administration (FDA) was on this issue and the answer was that marijuana was not safe or effective as medicine and should not be made available except for special research. That view has not changed. The World Health Organization and the United Nations Commission on Drugs oppose classifying marijuana as anything but an illicit substance ("Cannabis 'Safer than Alcohol and Tobacco" 2012).

Legislators influenced by anecdotal experiences from some constituents and by large campaign contributions from pro marijuana organizations and lobbyists should not decide what constitutes an acceptable medical product. That should be a scientific determination by the agency responsible by law for determining safe and effective medicines, the FDA.

Some believe that U.S. prisons are filled with unjustly incarcerated marijuana users. In fact, less than 1% of inmates in American prisons have been sent there solely for the use or possession of marijuana (*Who's Really in Prison for Marijuana?* 2005). There are thousands of marijuana arrests each month, but the offenders are not spending time in jail or prison unless there are more serious charges. Cook County Jail in Chicago houses approximately 9,500 prisoners every day; on a recent day a total of 90 were held overnight for possession of small amounts of marijuana, less than 40 others were out on electronic monitoring. Drug Courts hold great promise for drug offenders. Under Drug Court supervision, offenders can stay out of jail, be subject to drug testing which will clearly discourage use, and if after 6 months they stay clean and out of trouble, their arrest record can be expunged. The recidivism rate for our nation's 2,400 Drug Courts is 16%, one third the rate for offenders who do not go through this process (Rowan, Townsend, and Bhati 2003). Legislators should think about the value of intervention that comes with a criminal sanction so users can get treatment. Many drug users, including marijuana users, will not seek treatment unless compelled to do so.

Marijuana use has increased over the last decade as more states have enacted "medical" marijuana laws, but there are fewer individuals using illegal drugs today than the peak in the late 1970s. In 1978, approximately 25 million Americans used an illegal drug in the past month in a population of 225 million. In 2009, there were 22 million monthly users of illegal drugs in a population of 305 million U.S. citizens, constituting a drop in use from 11% of our population to 7% (National Survey on Drug Use and Health 2012).

Marijuana use, particularly for our young, is a serious problem. It may be tempting to try to find an easy answer, calling for legalization or decriminalization, but such a path would be a fool's choice. The leading admission category in public funded treatment centers in Los Angeles is for marijuana, not alcohol, with most for patients in their teens and early 20s. Keeping marijuana illegal and out of the hands of our young is in the public interest. Removing sanctions and disincentives to use will only contribute to higher health care costs, continued criminal activity, expanded dependency and compromised safety and productivity at work and at school.

References

"Cannabis 'Safer than Alcohol and Tobacco.'" BBC News. http://news.bbc.co.uk/2/hi/science/nature/58013.stm. Accessed on August 8, 2012.

"Health, Education, Safety Experts Join White House Drug Czar to Educate Parents About Risks of Youth Marijuana Use." U.S. Drug Enforcement Administration. http://www.justice.gov/dea/concern/ondcp_marijuana.html. Accessed on August 8, 2012.

Li, Mu-Chen, et al. 2011. "Marijuana Use and Motor Vehicle Crashes." *Epidemiological Reviews* 34(1): 65–72.

"'Medical' Marijuana." Save Our Society from Drugs. http://www.saveoursociety.org/our-issues/medical-marijuana. Accessed on August 8, 2012.

National Survey on Drug Use and Health. U.S. Department of Health and Human Services (Office of National Drug Control Policy). June 2, 2011. http://ofsubstance.gov/blogs/pushing_back/archive/2011/06/02/51896.aspx. Accessed on August 8, 2012.

"Results from the 2008 National Survey on Drug Use and Health: National Findings." Rockville, MD: Substance Abuse and Mental Health Services Administration, 2009.

Rowan, John, Wendy Townsend, and Avinash Singh Bhati. *Recidivism Rates for Drug Court Graduates: Nationally Based Estimates, Final Report.* https://www.ncjrs.gov/pdffiles1/201229.pdf, July 2003. Accessed on August 8, 2012.

Speaking Out against Drug Legislation. U.S. Drug Enforcement Administration. http://www.justice.gov/dea/demand/speak_out_101210.pdf. Accessed on August 8, 2012.

Who's Really in Prison for Marijuana? Office of National Drug Control Policy. http://www.prisonpolicy.org/scans/whos_in_prison_for_marij.pdf. Accessed on August 8, 2012.

Peter Bensinger is President and Chief Executive Officer of Bensinger, DuPont & Associates (BDA), a privately owned professional services company that provides a wide range of consultation, training, and employee assistance program services. He previously served as the Administrator of the U.S. Drug Enforcement Administration (DEA), as Director of the Illinois Department of Corrections, and as Chairman of the Illinois Youth Commission.

Is Marijuana Medicine? The Answer Is Yes, No, and Maybe

Kevin A. Sabet

Modern science has synthesized the marijuana plant's primary psychoactive ingredient THC into a pill form. This pill, dronabinol (or Marinol, its trade name) is sometimes prescribed for nausea and appetite stimulation. Another drug, Cesamet, mimics chemical structures similar to those found naturally in the plant.

But when most people think of medical marijuana these days, they don't think of a pill with an isolated component of marijuana, but rather the entire smoked, vaporized, or edible version of the whole marijuana plant. Rather than isolate active ingredients in the plant like we do with the opium plant when we create morphine, for example, many legalization proponents advocate vehemently for smoked marijuana to be used as a medicine. But the science on smoking any drug is clear: smoking especially highly potent whole marijuana is not a proper delivery method, nor do other delivery methods ensure a reliable dose. And while parts of the marijuana plant have medical value, the Institute of Medicine said in its landmark 1999 report: "Scientific data indicate the potential therapeutic value of cannabinoid drugs smoked marijuana, however, is a crude THC delivery system that also delivers harmful substances and should not be generally recommended" (Marijuana and Medicine: Assessing the Science Base 1999). It is not so unimaginable to think about other marijuana-based medications that might come to market very soon. Sativex, an oral mouth spray developed from a blend of two marijuana extracts (one strain is high in THC and the other in CBD, which counteracts THC's psychoactive effect), has already been approved in 10 countries and is in late stages of approval in the U.S. It is clear to anyone following this story that it is possible to develop marijuana-based medications in accordance with modern scientific standards, and many more such legitimate medications are just around the corner.

How Does Medical Marijuana Currently Work in the Various States?

At present in California, and in several other states, it is widely recognized that the reality of the "medical use" of marijuana is highly questionable. For payment of a small cash sum, almost anyone can obtain a physician's "recommendation" to purchase, possess, and use marijuana for alleged medical purposes. Indeed, numerous studies have shown that most customers of these dispensaries do not suffer from chronic, debilitating conditions such as HIV/AIDS or cancer (O'Connell and Bou Matar 2007; Nunberg et al. 2011). Both sides of the argument agree that this system has essentially legalized marijuana for recreational use, at least amongst those individuals able and willing to buy a recommendation (Lemon 2012). To date many pot dispensaries are mom and pop operations, though some act as multimillion-dollar, professional companies. A recent documentary on the Discovery Channel, which examined the practices of Harborside Health Center in Oakland, California, by its own admission, the largest marijuana dispensary "on the planet," the buds (which are distributed directly to member patients) are merely examined visually and with a microscope. The buds are also handled by employees who do not use gloves or face masks. Steve DeAngelo, Harborside's cofounder, states that they must "take it as it comes." The documentary noted that some plant material is tested by Steep Hill Laboratory, but there was no evidence that Steep Hill's instrumentation and techniques are "validated," that its operators are properly trained and educated, that its reference standards are accurate, and that its results are replicable by other laboratories. The City Council of Los Angeles recently voted unanimously to shutter dispensaries because of the increased crime, disorder, and drug use they have brought (Sabet, 2012).

What If We Rescheduled Marijuana?

In the wake of recent enforcement efforts by the Obama administration, the governors of Washington, Rhode Island, and Colorado have filed a petition with the Drug Enforcement Administration (DEA) to reschedule marijuana (Ingold 2012). Specifically, the petition asks the DEA to reclassify marijuana from Schedule I to Schedule II of the federal Controlled Substances Act (CSA). The governors contend that such rescheduling will eliminate the conflict between state and federal law and enable states to establish a "regulated and safe system to supply legitimate patients who may need medical cannabis."

The current petition takes a unique approach. It seeks to move marijuana to Schedule II "for medicinal purposes only." Marijuana advocacy organizations, such as the Marijuana Policy Project (MPP) and Americans for Safe Access (ASA), are urging other governors around the country to join the petition. The petition has garnered considerable publicity, but, as MPP acknowledges, "[r]escheduling is not a cure all" (Marijuana Policy Project 2012). This is an understatement. Indeed, it is not even a significant step in the direction that the governors, MPP, and ASA hope to move.

Part of the confusion over the actual significance of Schedule II status stems from a misunderstanding of the interrelated, but distinct, functions of the CSA and the Food, Drug, and

Cosmetic Act (FDCA). Under the FDCA, the FDA approves specific medical products produced by particular "innovator" (for branded products) or generic manufacturers. For example, oxycodone, an opioid, is in Schedule II. Specific products, such as OxyContin (an extended release form), are also in Schedule II. Physicians prescribe a specific branded or generic product, in a particular dose and dosage form. So until the FDA approves a smoked marijuana product, it cannot be prescribed or sold in "dispensaries" for medical use. And the FDA has been clear that smoked marijuana does not pass its rigorous approval standards (FDA Testimony 2009).

Imagine for a moment that the "medical marijuana" advocates were instead "medical opium" advocates and that various states passed laws decriminalizing (or affirmatively authorizing and regulating) the cultivation and distribution of opium plant material, i.e., opium latex or poppy straw. Even though opium latex and poppy straw are each in Schedule II, there would still be a conflict between such state laws and both the CSA and the FDCA. As a well-known drug reform advocacy website states: "If poppies are grown as sources for opiates, there is no question that it violates the CSA" (Opium Poppy: Legal Status 2012). Furthermore, physicians would not be authorized to prescribe, nor pharmacists to dispense, dried opium latex or poppy straw (Warning Letter 2010; Marketed Unapproved Drugs-Compliance Policy Guide). In order to be prescribed, a specific product containing opiates would have to pass muster in the FDA approval process. Therefore, the mere act of placing herbal marijuana in Schedule II would not make it available to patients nor address the conflict between state and federal law.

But Won't Rescheduling Allow for Research to Be Done?

No. Rescheduling is not necessary to make marijuana products available for research. A committee of the California Medical Association recently called for the rescheduling of marijuana "so it can be tested and regulated." However, it is not necessary for marijuana to be rescheduled in order for legitimate research to proceed. Schedule I status does not prevent a product from being tested and researched for potential medical use. Schedule I research certainly does go forward. In a recent pharmaceutical company-sponsored human clinical study investigating a product derived from marijuana extracts, the DEA registered approximately 30 research sites in the U.S. and also registered an importer to bring the product into the U.S. from the U.K., where it was manufactured (GW Pharmaceuticals 2006). And a quick search of NIH reporter reveals more than $14 million of current research going forward on marijuana and medicine. Research is happening.

What about Obtaining Marijuana for Research?

Researchers wishing to conduct studies with herbal/whole plant marijuana may obtain it from the National Institutes of Health (or import formulated extracts). Researchers who obtain grant funding from an institute of the National Institutes of Health (NIH), such as NIDA, can obtain marijuana for their study; researchers who are externally funded must undergo the equivalent of a grant review process (review of their study design by an expert committee of the Public Health Service) in order to obtain such marijuana at cost from NIDA. NIH (via the University of Mississippi's National Center for Natural Products Research) has the ability to produce standardized marijuana of varying THC potencies. Its cultivation area of five acres has been adequate to supply all marijuana-related studies to date. In theory, NCNPR could also produce marijuana extracts, or such products could be imported from outside the U.S. for research, as is currently the case with Sativex.

What Has Been the Result of Medical Marijuana in Various States on Drug Use Rates?

An in-depth examination of medical marijuana and its relationship to the explosion in use and users came in 2012 from five epidemiological researchers at Columbia University, and replicated again with another set of researchers (Cerda et al. 2011 and Wall et al. 2011). Using results from several large national surveys, they concluded that "residents of states with medical marijuana laws had higher odds or marijuana use and marijuana abuse/dependence than residents of states without such laws." States with medical marijuana laws also show much higher average marijuana use by adolescents, and lower perceptions of risk from use, than nonmedical pot states. This would seem to indicate that relaxed community norms about drug use contribute greatly to an increased prevalence of use and users, a situation resulting from the spread of an attitude that "if pot is medicine and is sanctioned by the state, then it must be safe to use by anyone."

Medical marijuana should really only be about bringing relief to the sick and dying, and it should be done in a responsible manner that formulates the active components of the drug in a non-smoked form that delivers a defined dose. However, in most states with medical marijuana laws, it has primarily become a license for the state-sanctioned use of a drug by most anyone who desires it. Developing marijuana-based medications through the FDA process is more likely to ensure that seriously ill patients, who are being supervised by their actual treating physicians, have access to safe and reliable products.

References

Cerda, M., et al. 2011. "Medical Marijuana Laws in 50 States: Investigating the Relationship between State Legalization of Medical Marijuana and Marijuana Use, Abuse and Dependence." *Drug and Alcohol Dependence.* http://www.columbia.edu/~dsh2/pdf/MedicalMarijuana.pdf. Accessed on July 26, 2012.

"FDA Testimony." http://www.fda.gov/NewsEvents/Testimony/ucm114741.htm. Accessed on July 26, 2012.

GW Pharmaceuticals. 2006. "Sativex Commences US Phase II/III Clinical Trial in Cancer Pain." http://www.fda.gov/

downloads/Drugs/GuidanceComplianceRegulatory
Information/Guidances/ucm070573.pdf. Accessed on
July 26, 2012.

Ingold, J. 2011. "Colorado Asks DEA To Reschedule
Marijuana." *Denver Post*. http://www.denverpost
.com/news/marijuana/ci_19636149. Accessed on January 20, 2012.

Lemon, Don. "Transcript of Don Lemon CNN Television
Show with Kevin Sabet and Allen St. Pierre." http://
transcripts.cnn.com/TRANSCRIPTS/0905/09/cnr.04
.html. Accessed on January 22, 2012.

Marijuana and Medicine: Assessing the Science Base. Institute
of Medicine, 1999. http://books.nap.edu/catalog.php?
record_id=6376. Accessed on January 20, 2012.

Marijuana Policy Project. "Message to Governors, Letter."
https://secure2.convio.net/mpp/site/Advocacy?
cmd=display&page=UserAction&id=1079. Accessed
on January 12, 2012.

"Marketed Unapproved Drugs-Compliance Policy Guide."
U.S. Food and Drug Administration. http://www.fda.gov/
downloads/Drugs/GuidanceComplianceRegulatory
Information/Guidances/ucm070290.pdf. Accessed on
January 20, 2012.

Nunberg, Helen, et al. 2011. "An Analysis of Applicants
Presenting to a Medical Marijuana Specialty Practice in
California." *Journal of Drug Policy Analysis* 4(1). http://www
.bepress.com/jdpa/vol4/iss1/art1. Accessed on January 20,
2012.

O'Connell, T. and C. B. Bou Matar. 2007. "Long Term
Marijuana Users Seeking Medical Cannabis in California
(2001 2007): Demographics, Social Characteristics, Patterns
of Cannabis and Other Drug Use of 4117 Applicants." *Harm
Reduction Journal*. http://www.harmreductionjournal.com/
content/4/1/1. Accessed on January 20, 2012.

"Opium Poppy: Legal Status." The Vaults of Erowid. http://
www.erowid.org/plants/poppy/poppy_law.shtml. Accessed
on January 20, 2012.

Sabet, Kevin. 2012. http://www.huffingtonpost.com/kevin-a
-sabet-phd/medical-marijuana-buyers-_b_1704230.html.
Accessed on January 20, 2012.

Wall, M., et al. 2011. "Adolescent Marijuana Use from 2002 to
2008: Higher in States with Medical Marijuana Laws, Cause
Still Unclear." *Annals of Epidemiology* 21(9): 714–716.

"Warning Letter." U.S. Food and Drug Administration.
June 28, 2010. http://www.fda.gov/ICECI/Enforcement
Actions/WarningLetters/ucm219984.htm. Accessed on
January 20, 2012.

*Kevin Sabet is Assistant Professor, University of Florida, Division of
Addiction Studies; Chief, Drug Policy Institute of University of
Florida; and President, Policy Solutions Lab.*

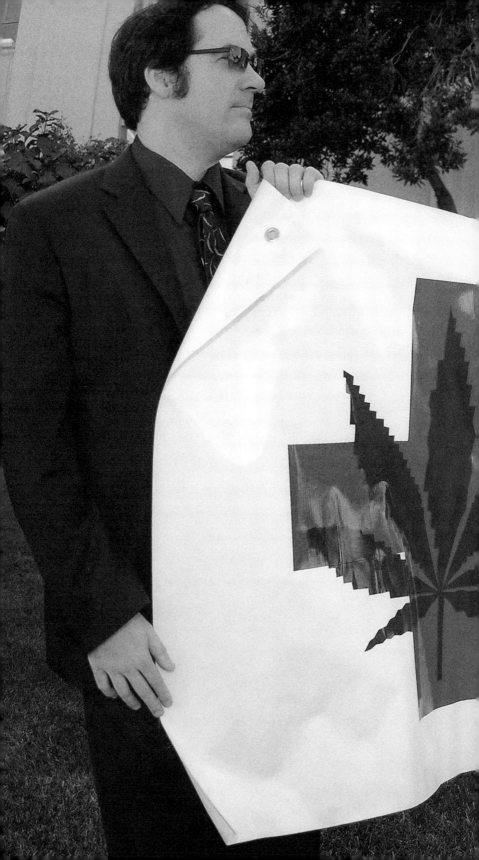

Introduction

This chapter contains brief sketches of individuals and organizations that are important in understanding the history of marijuana laws and policies in the United States and around the world. The number of such individuals and organizations is legion, and only some especially significant organizations and individuals, or those typical of other organizations and individuals, are included.

Americans for Safe Access

1322 Webster St., Suite 402
Oakland, CA 94612
Phone: (510) 251-1856
Fax: (510) 251-2036
E-mail: Info@SafeAccessNow.org
URL: http://www.safeaccessnow.org/
National Office
1806 Vernon St., N.W.
Washington, DC 20009

As of late 2012, eighteen states and the District of Columbia had adopted laws allowing the use of cannabis for medical purposes, with a number of other states considering such laws. (AP Photo/Chris Park)

Americans for Safe Access (ASA) was founded in 2002 by Steph Sherer, a woman with torticollis, a neurological movement disorder that causes a person's head to tilt to one side. The disorder is sometimes known colloquially as "wry neck." It is accompanied by pain, inflammation, and muscle spasms that may be relieved by the use of marijuana. Sherer founded ASA for the purpose of educating the general public about the medical uses of cannabis and combating efforts by the U.S. Drug Enforcement Administration (DEA) to prevent the use of marijuana for medical purposes in places where state law permits such use. ASA claims to be "the largest national member-based organization of patients, medical professionals, scientists and concerned citizens promoting safe and legal access to cannabis for therapeutic use and research." At the time that Sherer founded ASA, there were only 11 marijuana dispensaries in the United States, all of which were operating illegally at the time because no state had yet legalized the use of marijuana for therapeutic purposes. As of 2012, there are more than 500 marijuana dispensaries in California alone, and an estimated 2,100 dispensaries and other facilities where medical marijuana is distributed throughout the nation.

ASA has developed a multifaceted program to achieve its objective of ensuring safe and legal access to anyone who needs the substance for therapeutic or research purposes. Some elements of that program are:

- The Medical Cannabis Advocate's Training Center, at which individuals are trained about the history and science of marijuana as a therapeutic agent and are taught the skills needed to work effectively within the political system to accomplish ASA goals.

- The Medical Cannabis Think Tank and Policy Shop, which studies current political and legislative developments with regard to therapeutic marijuana and offer information and advice to policymakers and legislators on relevant topics.

- The Sick and Tired Campaign, designed to place increasing pressure on President Barack Obama to move forward more rapidly on efforts to make medical marijuana legal and available, including a petition drive to the president, an Obama Report Card outlining progress (or lack of it) the president has made, and participation in the Coalition to Reschedule Cannabis.

- The Federal Advocacy Project, run out of the Washington office of ASA, attempts to influence policymakers and legislators at all levels about the objectives of the safe marijuana movement.

- The California Campaign for Safe Access, which focuses specifically on the largest state in which medical marijuana has been legalized, dealing with patient's rights, education about the medical marijuana law in the state, and efforts to ensure that the law is implemented properly.

- The Raid Center, which is a carefully organized, specific program designed to help individuals and organizations whose activities have been subjected to raids by the DEA or other law enforcement agencies.

- The Take a Close Look: Cannabis Is Medicine program that promotes better understanding about the medical role of cannabis in treating a wide variety of disorders.

- The Patient's Rights Project, which deals directly with individuals who use marijuana therapeutically, explaining to them on a one-to-one basis what their rights are with regard to medical cannabis.

- The Community Support Project, an ambitious effort to provide all stakeholders in the medical marijuana community with the information and guidance they need to function effectively in their specific roles, with special programs for patients, clinicians, and medical advocates.

- State campaigns, in which the resources and skills available among ASA staff are made available to medical marijuana efforts in individual states across the nation.

- The Welcome to ASA 3.0 project that was designed to inform patients and the general public about three new pieces of legislation recently introduced into the U.S. Congress, H.R. 1983, the Medical Marijuana Patient Protection Act; H.R. 1984, the Small Business Banking Improvement Act of 2011; and H.R. 1985, the Small Business Tax Equity Act of 2011.

An important insight into the work that ASA does is its annual listing of major accomplishments. For 2011, that list included such items as:

- Gave stronger voice to the needs of patients in the national debate over medical marijuana.

- Won litigation against the California Highway Patrol's practice of confiscating a person's medical marijuana when stopped for nonrelated violations.

- Represented individuals who had lost property as a result of federal action against state medical marijuana laws.

- Established a new office in Washington, DC, with the sole objective of working on medical marijuana issues, the only one of its kind in the city.

- Worked with elected officials and community members to develop and pass new medical marijuana laws and to ensure proper enforcement of existing laws.

- Provided peer counseling, legal training, raid response, media training, and other services to patients and providers.

- Published more than a million legal manuals, more than 2 million Know Your Rights wallet cards, and hundreds of thousands of training manuals.

- Orchestrated more than 200 protests to DEA raids at medical dispensaries, using social networking tools to achieve maximum effect.

- Conducted hundreds of training sessions for patients, providers, attorneys, clinicians, and advocates.

ASA annually publishes a wide variety of position statements, reports, background papers, and other documents on various aspects of the medical marijuana issue. Among the publications currently available are the policy statements "Cannabis as Medicine," "Patients' Bill of Rights," "Reclassifying Medical Cannabis," "President Obama's Policy on Medical Cannabis," "Who Should Qualify as a Patient?", "Medical Cannabis Research," "Patient Cultivation," "Medical Cannabis and Genetic Engineering," and "Recognition and Regulation of Distribution Centers."

Harry J. Anslinger (1892–1975)

Anslinger was appointed the first commissioner of the Federal Bureau of Narcotics when it was established in 1930. He held that office for 32 years, one of the longest tenures of any federal official in modern history. He was consistently a strong advocate for severe penalties against the manufacture, distribution, sale, and use of certain drugs, especially marijuana.

Harry Jacob Anslinger was born in Altoona, Pennsylvania, on May 20, 1892, to Robert J. and Rosa Christiana Fladt Anslinger, immigrants from Switzerland and Germany, respectively. Without completing high school, Anslinger attended the Altoona Business College before taking a job with the Pennsylvania Railroad. He received a leave of absence from the railway that allowed him to matriculate at Pennsylvania State College (now Pennsylvania State University), where he received his two-year associate degree in engineering and business management. He then returned to a full-time job at the railroad.

When World War I broke out, Anslinger was rejected for active service because of a childhood accident that had left him blind in one eye. Instead, he was accepted for volunteer service at the War Department in Washington, DC, where he was made assistant to the Chief of Inspection of Equipment. He remained at the War Department for only a year before being transferred to the State Department, where his fluency in German was a greater asset. His first overseas assignment at State was to the U.S. mission in the Hague, Netherlands, in 1918, where he was made special liaison to the deposed king of Germany, Wilhelm II. Three years later, Anslinger was transferred to the U.S. mission in Hamburg, Germany, and then, three years later, he was transferred again, this time to the U.S. mission in La Guaira, Venezuela.

In 1926, Anslinger received yet another assignment, this time to Nassau, in the British Bahamas. His job in Nassau was to try to reduce the flow of liquor from the Bahamas to the United States, following the adoption of the Prohibition amendment to the U.S. Constitution in 1920. At the time, the Bahamas were one of the major venues for the shipment of illegal alcohol to the United States. Anslinger's work in this post was so impressive that the U.S. Treasury asked the State Department to transfer him to its own offices in Washington, DC. His first job at Treasury was as chief of the Division of Foreign Control. That post allowed him to become active in the international war against illegal drugs, a war of major concern to the United States but of relatively little concern to most other countries in the world. As official representative of the United States, Anslinger attended the Conference on Suppression of Smuggling in London in 1926; the Conference on Suppression of Smuggling in Paris in 1927; and the International Congress against Alcoholism in Antwerp in 1928. In all of these settings, Anslinger worked aggressively to promote an American agenda for much stronger legislative and regulatory controls over the production, transport, and use of narcotics, including marijuana.

In 1929, Anslinger was promoted to assistant commissioner in the U.S. Bureau of Prohibition. He held that position only briefly before being selected as the first commissioner of the newly created Federal Bureau of Narcotics in 1930. He began his assignment at the bureau at a time when state and federal officials were debating the need (or lack of need) for regulations of hemp and marijuana. Both hemp and marijuana are obtained from plants in the genus *Cannabis*, the former with many important industrial applications, and the latter used almost exclusively as a recreational drug. Historians have discussed the motivations that may have driven Anslinger's attitudes about the subject, but his actions eventually demonstrated a strong opposition to the growing, processing, distribution, and use of all products of the cannabis plant. He was instrumental in formulating federal policies and laws against such use that developed during the 1930s. Throughout his career, he also continued his efforts to influence the direction of international drug policies, always working for more severe penalties in drug trafficking and use. In this effort, he served as co-observer at the League of Nations Opium Advisory Commission between 1932 and 1939, as a delegate to the International Conference for Suppression of Illicit Traffic in Narcotic Drugs of the League of Nations in 1936, and as U.S. representative to the Commission on Narcotic Drugs of the United Nations in 1952.

Anslinger has long been criticized for the extremes with which he pursued his campaign against drugs and his use of racist and sexist themes in that campaign. At one time or another, for example, he wrote that:

- "There are 100,000 total marijuana smokers in the US, and most are Negroes, Hispanics, Filipinos and entertainers. Their Satanic music, jazz and swing, result from marijuana usage. This marijuana causes white women to seek sexual relations with Negroes, entertainers and any others."

- "Marihuana influences Negroes to look at white people in the eye, step on white men's shadows and look at a white woman twice."

- "Reefer makes darkies think they're as good as white men."

Anslinger remained in his post until 1970, staying on even after his seventieth birthday until a replacement was found. He then served two more years as U.S. representative to the UN Narcotic Drugs Convention. By the end of his tenure with the convention, he was blind and suffered from both angina and an enlarged prostate. He died in Hollidaysburg, Pennsylvania, on November 14, 1975, of heart failure. Although little definitive information is available, Anslinger apparently earned his LL.B. (bachelor of laws degree) from the Washington College of Law in 1930, and was later awarded an honorary LL.D. (doctor of laws) degree from the University of Maryland (date unknown). Among his many awards were the Proctor Gold Medal, Alumni Recognition Award of American University, distinguished alumnus award of Pennsylvania State University, Remington Medal, and the Alexander Hamilton Medal. He was the coauthor of two major books, *The Traffic in Narcotics* (with William F. Tompkins; Funk & Wagnalls, 1953) and *The Murderers: The Story of the Narcotic Gangs* (with Will Ousler; Farrar, Strauss, and Cudahy, 1961).

Drug Free America Foundation, Inc.
5999 Central Ave., Suite 301
Saint Petersburg, FL 33710
Phone: (727) 828-0211
Fax: (727) 828-0212
E-mail: webmaster@dfaf.org.
URL: http://www.dfaf.org/

Drug Free America Foundation, Inc. (DFAF) is a 501(c)(3) nonprofit organization that, according to its mission statement, is "committed to developing, promoting and sustaining global strategies, policies and laws that will reduce illegal drug use, drug addiction, drug-related injury and death." The organization was founded by Mr. and Mrs. Mel Sembler in 1995. Mr. Sembler was chairman of the board of the Sembler Company, a developer and manager of shopping centers. He also served as U.S. ambassador to Italy and to Australia and Nauru. In the DFAF 2010 annual report, Mrs. Sembler is listed as founder and chair of the organization.

Mr. and Mrs. Sembler originally founded the organization known as Straight, Inc., in 1976, as a nonprofit drug treatment program that claims to have treated more than 12,000 young people with substance abuse problems in eight cities in the United States. Straight was long the subject of intense scrutiny for alleged abusive practices used in its drug treatment programs. It later changed its name to Straight Foundation, Inc., and spun off a number of drug treatment programs such as The Seed, Kids Helping Kids, Pathway Family Center, Life, Growing Together, KIDS (of various cities and regions), SAFE, and Alberta Adolescent Recovery Center (AARC). Drug Free America Foundation is reputed to be one of the Straight spinoffs. The DFAF website makes little or no mention of this alleged connection.

Most of DFAF's work is carried out through six divisions:

- The Institute on Global Drug Policy is an alliance of physicians, scientists, attorneys, and drug specialists who advocate for the adoption of public policies that curtail the use of illicit and misuse of licit drugs and alcohol. A major activity of the institute is cosponsorship of the *Journal of Global Drug Policy and Practice* with another division of DFAF, the International Scientific and Medical Forum on Drug Abuse. Relatively little information is available online about the organization, membership, or activities of the institute. In a statement announcing formation of the division, its mission was described as "creating and strengthening international laws that hold drug users and dealers criminally accountable for their actions. It will vigorously promote treaties and agreements that provide clear penalties to individuals who buy, sell or use harmful drugs. It will push for a uniform legal requirement that marijuana and other addictive drugs must meet the same scientific standards as other drugs to be deemed therapeutic for medical conditions."

- The International Scientific and Medical Forum on Drug Abuse is described by DFAF as a "brain trust" of researchers and physicians concerned about substance abuse who have an interest in dispelling incorrect depictions of the consequences of drug use among the general public. The division is a cosponsor of the *Journal of Global Drug Policy and Practice* with The Institute on Global Drug Policy.

• The International Task Force on Strategic Drug Policy is a network of professionals in the field of substance abuse and community leaders who work together to develop and implement drug reduction principles around the world. The task force convenes meetings in cooperation with other divisions of the DFAF to train individuals in methods of drug reduction principles. The task force reports having held eight such conferences of about 60 to 130 individuals since 2001 in locations such as London, Buenos Aires, Tampa, and Guayaquil, Ecuador.

• The Drug Prevention Network of the Americas (DPNA) is a cooperative effort of nongovernmental agencies in North, South, and Central America working to reduce demand for illegal substances through conferences, training seminars, and Internet communications.

• Students Taking Action Not Drugs (STAND) is a student-based organization whose goal it is to distribute on campuses accurate scientific information about the effects of taking illegal drugs.

• National Drug-Free Workplace Alliance (NDWA) is a division attempting to develop drug free work environments in the state of Florida and, working with other agencies and organizations, throughout the United States.

The organization's website provides its views on a broad array of drug topics, including marijuana, overcoming addiction, prescription drug abuse, drug policy, drug testing, prevention of substance abuse, and international drug policy. Associated with each topic is a PDF file or other attachment that provides more detail on the subject such as PDF files on federal and state laws dealing with medical marijuana, "the truth" about marijuana, and how to get rich by suing a doctor who prescribes marijuana for medical purposes. The organization's website also lists the Otto and Connie Moulton Library for Drug Prevention, which contains more than 2,100 books and other media dealing with substance abuse issues, which visitors to the site are invited to access. In addition to three position statements on substance abuse (on harm reduction, student drug testing, and medical marijuana), DFAF also offers a small number of DVDs dealing with substance abuse issues, including "True Compassion: About Marijuana," "Real View Mirror: Looking at Your Future, Leaving the Drug Culture Behind," "In Focus: A Clear Message about Drugs," and "Deadly Indifference: The Price of Ignoring the Youth Drug Epidemic."

Drug Policy Alliance

70 W. 36th St., 16th Floor
New York, NY 10018
Phone: (212) 613-8020
Fax: (212) 613-8021
URL: http://www.drugpolicy.org/
Email: nyc@drugpolicy.org

The Drug Policy Alliance (DPA) was created in July 2000 as a result of the merger of the Lindesmith Center (TLC) and the Drug Policy Foundation (DPF). The Lindesmith Center, in turn, had been formed in 1994 as a think tank for the consideration of alternatives to existing policies and practices for dealing with drug issues, while the Drug Policy Foundation had been established in 1987 as an organization established to work for drug reform, largely through the provision of grants to advance further studies on drug policies. The DPA now claims to be "the world's leading drug policy reform organization of people who believe the war on drugs is doing more harm than good." The organization currently claims to have nearly 30,000 members, with an additional 70,000 individuals receiving its online e-newsletter and action alerts.

DPA organizes its work under the rubric of about a half-dozen major issues: reforming marijuana laws, fighting injustice, reducing drug harm, protecting youth, defending personal liberty, and making economic sense. Each of these general topics is further divided into more specific issues. The reforming marijuana laws topic, for example, covers issues such as developing a legal regulatory market for marijuana, helping individuals who have been arrested for marijuana possession, and providing information about the potential health and social effects of marijuana use. The topic of protecting youth is further divided into efforts to deal with drug testing in schools and zero-tolerance policies in some school districts, as well as providing information and materials on "reality-based" drug education. The making economic sense topic deals in more detail with subjects such as problems of supply and demand for marijuana, the problem of drug prohibition and violence, and the economic benefits of legalizing and taxing the sale of marijuana.

An important part of the DPA efforts on behalf of marijuana issue is a series of Action Alerts through which members and friends of the association are encouraged to contact legislators, administrative officials, and other stakeholders about specific issues of concern to the organization. During 2012, for example, DPA sponsored Action Alerts directed to members of the U.S. Senate about protection of medical marijuana patients, a campaign to influence President Barack Obama to work harder to protection of medical marijuana patients, efforts to lobby members of the U.S. Congress to end criminalization of marijuana use and possession, and a campaign to encourage Congress to reduce federal spending on the enforcement of existing marijuana laws.

The Drug Policy Alliance publishes a number of reports, fact sheets, and other print and electronic materials on the topic of marijuana legalization. Members receive the tri-annual newsletter the *Ally*, which provides information on the organization's current activities and successes. Other publications include *Safety First: A Reality-Based Approach to Teens and Drugs*, a tool designed to help parents evaluate and discuss strategies for protecting teenagers from drug abuse; *Crime and Punishment in New Jersey: The Criminal Code and Public Opinion on Sentencing*, a report on the legal status of marijuana in that state; *Drug Courts Are Not the Answer: Toward a Health-Centered Approach to Drug Use*, an analysis of existing laws on marijuana possession; *Overdose: A National Crisis Taking Root in Texas*, a report on the growing number of overdose deaths in that state and the United States; *Arresting Latinos for Marijuana in California: Possession Arrests in 33 Cities, 2006–08*, a report on the special risk faced by Latinos in California for marijuana offenses; and *Healing a Broken System: Veterans Battling Addiction and Incarceration*, which deals with the special problems of marijuana use faced by veterans returning from service in Iraq and Afghanistan.

On its website, DPA also provides an excellent resource that deals with drug facts. Some of the topics covered on this page include fundamental facts about marijuana and other drugs, some new solutions for dealing with the nation's drug problems, the relevance of federal and state drug laws for individuals, a summary of individual rights in connection with existing drug laws, statistical information about the nation's war on drugs, and drug laws around the world.

European Monitoring Centre for Drugs and Drug Addiction

Cais do Sodré
1249-289 Lisbon
Portugal
Phone: +351-211-21-02-00
Fax: +351-218-13-17-11
E-mail: info@emcdda.europa.eu
URL: http://www.emcdda.europa.eu/index.cfm

The concept of an all-European agency to deal with the growing problem of substance abuse on the continent was first proposed by French President Georges Pompidou in the late 1960s. That idea languished for about two decades before it was raised once more in 1989 by French President François Mitterrand in 1989. Mitterrand suggested a seven-step program that would involve establishing a common method for analyzing drug addiction in the European states, harmonizing national policies for substance abuse, strengthening controls and improving cooperation among states, finding ways of implementing the 1988 UN Convention Against Illicit Traffic in Narcotic Drugs and Psychotropic Substances, coordinating policies and practices between producing and consuming countries, developing a common policy dealing with drug-related money laundering, and designating a single individual in each country responsible for anti-drug actions within that country.

Mitterrand's suggestion led to a series of actions within the European Community that eventually resulted, in 1993, in the creation of the European Monitoring Centre for Drugs and Drug Addiction (EMCDDA) under Council Regulation (EEC) number 302/93. The general administrative structure was established the following year, consisting of an executive director, a management board, and a scientific committee. The management board is the primary decision-making body for EMCDDA. It meets at least once a year and is composed of one representative from each member state of the European Union (EU), two representatives from the European Commission, and two representatives from the European Parliament. The board adopts an annual work program and a three-year work program that guides the organization's day-to-day operations. The three-year program is developed with input from a wide variety of sources, including the general public (through the organization's website). The 2010 to 2012 program focused on topics such as refining methodologies to allow better identification and monitoring of new and established substances; developing a framework for monitoring illegal drug supply, drug markets, and drug-related crimes; improving methods for estimating and describing dependence and drug problems in populations using nonopiate drugs; and developing guidelines and good practice standards for interventions and the development and dissemination of quality standards.

The scientific committee consists of 15 members appointed by the management board for the purpose of advising the board on scientific issues related to substance abuse. The first meeting of the management board was held in April 1994 at its Lisbon headquarters, where its administrative offices remain today. Much of the work of EMCDDA takes place within eight units of the scientific committee. The eight units focus on prevalence, consequences, and data management; supply reduction and new trends; interventions, best practice, and scientific partners; policy, evaluation, and content coordination; Reitox and international cooperation; and communication; information and communication technology; and administration. Reitox is the name given to a network of human and computer links among the 27 nations that make up the EMCDDA operation.

The EMCDDA website is one of the richest resources available on nearly every aspect of substance abuse issues in the world. It contains information on a wide variety of topics such as health consequences (deaths and mortality, infectious diseases, treatment demand, and viral hepatitis); prevalence and epidemiology (general population surveys, drug trends in youth, problem drug use, key indicators, and wastewater analysis); best practice (prevention, treatment, harm reduction, standards and guidelines), Exchange on Drug Demand Reduction Action (EDDRA), and Evaluation Instruments Bank (EIB); drug profiles (amphetamine, barbiturates, benzodiazepines, BZP and other piperazines, cannabis, cocaine and crack, fentanyl, hallucinogenic mushrooms, heroin, khat, LSD, MDMA, methamphetamine, *Salvia divinorum*, synthetic cannabinoids and "Spice," synthetic cathinones, synthetic cocaine derivatives, and volatile substances); health and social interventions (harm reduction, prevention of drug use, social reintegration, and treatment of drug use); policy and law (EU policy and law, laws, and public expenditure); new drugs and trends (action on new drugs); supply and supply reduction (interventions against drug supply, interventions against diversion of chemical precursors, interventions against money laundering activities, supply reduction, markets, and crime and supply reduction indicators); resources by drug (cannabis thematic page, cocaine and crack thematic page, and opioids and heroin thematic page); drugs and society (crime, driving, social exclusion, women and gender issues, and young people); and science and research (addiction medicine, neuroscience, and research in Europe).

Over the decades, EMCDDA has produced a plethora of publications on virtually every imaginable aspect of substance abuse, including all possible topics related to cannabis. Among the 2011 publications are National Reports for the 27 EU countries plus Croatia and Turkey; selected issues reports on "Guidelines for the Treatment of Drug Dependence: A European Perspective," "Mortality Related to Drug Use in Europe," and "Cost and Financing of Drug Treatment Services in Europe;" "Summary Report from EMCDDA Trendspotter Meeting 18–19 October 2011" (reports of scientific Research); "Pilot Study on Wholesale Drug Prices in Europe" (a thematic paper); and "ECDC and EMCDDA Guidance: Prevention and Control of Infectious Diseases among People Who Inject Drugs" (a joint publication with the European Centre for Disease Prevention and Control). One of EMCDDA's most valuable publications is its annual *General Report of Activities*, which describes in some detail the work undertaken and completed by the organization during the preceding year. The publication is available online at http://www.emcdda.europa.eu/attachements.cfm/att _136906_EN_TDAB11001ENN_FINAL_Web.pdf.

Barney Frank (1940–)

Frank is a long-serving (since 1981) member of the U.S. House of Representatives from the Fourth Congressional District of Massachusetts. He is widely regarded as one of the most liberal members of both the House and of the Democratic Party. He is perhaps best remembered for his legislative efforts during the economic downturn that began in 2006. He spearheaded passage of legislation that led to the creation of the Troubled Asset Relief Program (TARP) in 2008, which allowed the U.S. Treasury to buy up bad mortgage securities. In 2010, he was one of the two major cosponsors (with Senator Christopher Dodd, D-CT) of a bill enacting regulatory reform of the nation's financial structure. Frank was also lead sponsor of a number of bills to reform the nation's marijuana laws, essentially aimed at reducing or eliminating fines and penalties for the use of marijuana for personal purposes. During his tenure, Frank has sponsored and cosponsored a number of bills designed to decriminalize marijuana and to authorize the use of marijuana for medical purposes. Among these bills were the States' Rights to Medical Marijuana Act of 2001 (H.R. 2592), the Personal Use of Marijuana by Responsible Adults Act of 2008 (HR 5843; reintroduced in 2009 as H.R. 2943), the States' Medical Marijuana Patient Protection Act of 2011 (H.R. 1983), and the Ending Federal Marijuana Prohibition Act of 2011 (H.R. 2306). Frank announced in December 2011 that he would not run for re-election in 2012. He cited as one reason for his decision the increasingly polarized political debates taking place in the Congress. Political observers noted that a redistricting plan produced a dramatically different population for his Fourth District that, although likely still to be strongly Democratic in orientation, would have required a significant effort on Frank's part to learn more about his new constituents' political viewpoints.

Barney Frank was born Barnett Frank on March 31, 1940, in Bayonne, New Jersey, to Samuel and Elsie (née Golush) Frank. Samuel Frank operated a truck stop in Jersey City, which reputedly had connections to crime that led to his incarceration in prison for a year. After graduating from Bayonne High School in 1957, Frank matriculated at Harvard College, from which he graduated in 1962. (He had taken a year off to deal with family affairs upon his father's death, a period during which his father's Mafia friends were "very helpful.") Frank then enrolled in the PhD program in government at Harvard but left the program in 1968 to become chief assistant for Boston mayor Kevin White. Although Frank eventually earned his law degree from Harvard in 1977, he had set his path on a role in politics by joining White's staff. After three years with the mayor, he joined the staff of Congressman Michael J. Harrington, Democratic representative from the Massachusetts's Sixth District, as administrative assistant.

After a year with Representative Harrington, Frank ran for and won a seat in the Massachusetts House of Representatives from Boston's Back Bay District. He also immediately made a name for himself crusading for liberal approaches to solving social problems in Boston. He was easily elected to three more terms in the Massachusetts House. In addition to his position in the Massachusetts legislature, Frank taught part time at the Harvard University John F. Kennedy School of Government, at the University of Massachusetts at Boston, and at Boston University. He was admitted to the Massachusetts bar in 1979.

A somewhat unusual opportunity presented itself to Frank in 1979 when Pope John Paul II decreed that members of the Roman Catholic clergy were not allowed to hold political office, thereby making it impossible for the sitting member of the U.S. House of Representatives for Massachusetts's Fourth District, Father Robert Drinan, from continuing in office. Frank ran for the office and won by a vote of 52 percent to 48 percent. Two years later, Frank anticipated an even more difficult challenge when he was paired with sitting Congresswoman Margaret Heckler in the newly drawn Fourth District. Frank won the election by 20 percentage points. It was the closest election he was to experience during the rest of his career.

Frank has written two books, *Speaking Frankly: What's Wrong with the Democrats and How to Fix It* (1992, Crown Books) and *Frank Talk: The Wit and Wisdom of Barney Frank* (2006, iUniverse), as well as a number of legislative reports produced by the Congressional Digest Corporation such as *Affordable Housing: Addressing the Basic Needs of Low-income*

Families: Should the House Approve H.R. 2895, the National Affordable Housing Trust Fund Act? (2007), *Executive Compensation: Regulating the Pay of Top Corporate Managers— Should the House Pass H.R. 3269, the Corporate and Financial Institution Compensation Fairness Act?* (2009), and *Helping Homeowners: Mortgage Foreclosures and Bankruptcy Reform: Should the House Pass H.R. 1106, the Helping Families Save Their Homes Act?*

Jon Gettman (1957–)

Gettman has long been active in the campaign to have marijuana rescheduled under provisions of the Controlled Substances Act of 1970 (CSA) from its current listing as a schedule I substance to a less restrictive status. A schedule I substance is so listed because (1) it has a high potential for abuse, (2) the substance has no currently accepted medical use in treatment in the United States, and (3) there is a lack of accepted safety for use of the substance under medical supervision. The act makes it illegal for any person, except with special authorization, (1) to manufacture, distribute, dispense, or possess with intent to manufacture, distribute, or dispense, the substance or (2) to create, distribute, or dispense, or possess with intent to distribute or dispense, a counterfeit of the scheduled substance. For more than a decade, Gettman has been a leader of the Coalition for Rescheduling Cannabis, a group of organizations and individuals seeking to have marijuana listed under a less restrictive CSA schedule. Members of the coalition include the American Alliance for Medical Cannabis, Americans for Safe Access, California NORML, the Drug Policy Forum of Texas, *High Times* magazine, the Los Angeles Cannabis Resource Center, NORML, the Oakland Cannabis Buyers Cooperative, and Patients Out of Time.

Jon Gettman was born on August 20, 1957. He attended the Catholic University of America, from which he received his BA in anthropology in 1985; the American University

(Washington, DC), which awarded him his MS in justice (with a specialization in drug policy) in 1992; and George Mason University, where he received his PhD in public policy (specialization: regional economic development) in 2000. While still a young man, from 1973 to 1980, Gettman worked for the Stone Age Trading Company in wholesale and retail management. He then became involved in the effort to have marijuana use legalized in the United States, serving as policy analyst, business manager, director of communications, president, and national director of NORML from 1981 to 1993. In 1994, he left NORML to work on his own. He has been research analyst, program manager, expert witness, and writer and columnist for public policy, business, legal, and editorial clients. In these roles, he has testified in important cannabis-related cases, including *United States v. Phillip Schmoll, Commonwealth of Pennsylvania v. Ryan Free, United States v. Timothy Perry, Commonwealth of Virginia v. Michael Firth, Commonwealth of Pennsylvania v. James Almquist, Commonwealth of Virginia v. David May*, and *Commonwealth of Virginia v. Brad Gillies*. Gettman has also appeared before state and federal legislative bodies, including the House/Senate Special Subcommittee of Agriculture, the House Committee of Agriculture of the Virginia legislature, and the Senate Judiciary Committee of the Alaska legislature. In addition to his freelance work as a consultant, Gettman has held other work positions such as program development, research analysis, and project management for Mouncey & Company, Waterford, Virginia; instructor at the College of Southern Maryland, La Plata, Maryland, and volunteer resource person for the Loudoun County, Virginia, Task Force to Propose a Rural Economic Development Plan. Gettman has also taught the following classes: Management in a Technological Society (University of Maryland University College); Public Administration (Shepherd University); American History to 1865 (College of Southern Maryland); and Introduction to Public Administration (College of Southern Maryland). Between 2003 and 2005 and from 2008 to the present, Gettman has also been senior research fellow at the George Mason School of Public Policy.

Gettman has written and spoken extensively about the reclassification of cannabis in the United States. Among his print articles are "Marijuana Arrests in Massachusetts," "Marijuana Treatment Admissions," "Marijuana Use in the United States," "Lost Taxes and Other Costs of Marijuana Laws," "Marijuana Production in the United States" (all *Bulletin of Cannabis Reform*); "Marijuana and the Controlled Substances Act" (*Journal of Cannabis Therapeutics*); and "Decriminalizing Marijuana" (*American Behavioral Scientist*). Among his conference presentations are "Medical Cannabis and the Public Policy Process" (Fifth National Clinical Conference on Cannabis Therapeutics); "Medical Cannabis and the Public Policy Process" (Fourth National Clinical Conference on Cannabis Therapeutics); "Dynamic Portfolio Variance Analysis and the Study of Regional Economic Instability" (Southern Regional Science Association); "Crimes of Indiscretion: Marijuana Arrests in the United States" (2005 Conference of the National Organization for the Reform of Marijuana Laws); "DEA Rescheduling Report" (Third National Clinical Conference on Cannabis Therapeutics); "Personal Use v. Distribution of Cannabis" (Fall Meeting and Seminar of the Virginia College of Criminal Defense Attorneys); "Domestic and International Regulations: Cannabis" (American Academy of Pain Management, 12th Annual Clinical Meeting); "Marijuana and Drug Treatment: An Introduction" (Saving Our Children From Abusive Drug Treatment conference); and "Science and the End of Marijuana Prohibition" (12th International Conference on Drug Policy Reform).

Hemp Industries Association

P.O. Box 575
Summerland, CA 93067
Phone: (707) 874-3648
Fax: (707) 874-3648

E-mail: info@thehia.org
URL: http://thehia.org/

The Hemp Industries Association (HIA) is a federally chartered 501(c)(6) nonprofit organization representing the hemp industry in the United States, Canada, and other countries, including Australia, China, Mexico, the Netherlands, New Zealand, and the United Kingdom. The organization was formed in 1992 to work for fair and equitable treatment of hemp, a material produced from the cannabis plant with a very low (usually less than 1 percent) concentration of Δ^9-tetrahydrocannabinol (THC), the compound responsible for the psychoactive effects associated with the ingestion of marijuana. The mission statement of the organization lists the following goals:

• Educate the general public about the qualities of hemp that make it useful for a variety of consumer products.
• Facilitate the exchange of information among all stakeholders in the hemp industry, including agriculturists, processors, manufacturers, distributors, and retailers.
• Ensure the integrity of hemp products.
• Advocate for and promote socially responsible and environmentally sound business practices.

As of 2012, the organization had about 130 members representing virtually every conceivable phase of the hemp industry. Some examples of HIA members and the products and services they offer include:

• AZIDA: Body care products
• Coalition for Hemp Awareness: A consulting firm
• Nature's Path Organic Foods: Food products
• BACH/Creative Expressions: Books and periodicals
• Cannabag: Bags
• Dr. Bronner's Magic Soaps: Body care and food products

- Hemp Traders: Textiles, fabric, and yarns
- Nutiva: Books, periodicals, food products, seed oil, seeds, and grain
- Satori Movement/Creation Skateboards: Apparel, accessories, and skateboards
- Son's Development and Green Building Supplies: Building materials
- Steve's Cat Toys: Pet accessories and animal care products
- Ultra Oil for Pets: Animal care products and seed oil
- Concord Minutemen Solutions Group: Consulting, lobbying, promoting, and marketing
- Natureflections: Paper products
- Hempcore: Sports equipment
- Hemphasis magazine: Books and periodicals

(On its website at http://www.thehia.org/products.html, the organization lists more than 100 products made from hemp that are produced and sold by its members.)

One of HIA's most important accomplishments was defeat of a 2001 effort by the U.S. Drug Enforcement Administration (DEA) to include hemp under schedule I of the Controlled Substances Act of 1970 (CSA), a category under which another cannabis product, marijuana, is currently listed. Substances listed under schedule I are regarded as (1) having a high potential for abuse, (2) having no currently accepted medical use in treatment in the United States, and (3) lacking safe use under medical supervision. The DEA argued that it had the authority to list hemp as a schedule I substance because in almost all cases, the fibers and oils made from hemp contain greater than zero concentrations of THC. Granted that those concentrations are very low, the DEA said, they are still measurable and, therefore, capable of being listed under schedule I under the CSA. The Hemp Industries Association brought suit against the DEA, claiming that the agency had gone beyond the provisions laid down by the CSA. The association was funded and supported in this effort by one of its best known and economically successful members, known at the time as ALL-ONE-GOD-FAITH, Inc., doing business as (and much better known to the public as) Dr. Bronner's Magic Soaps, and joined by a number of other hemp interests, including Atlas Corporation; Nature's Path Foods USA, Inc.; Hemp Oil Canada, Inc.; Hempzels, Inc.; Kenex Ltd.; Tierra Madre, LLC; Ruth's Hemp Foods, Inc.; and the Organic Consumers Association. Plaintiffs were eventually successful in their complaint, with the Ninth Circuit Court of Appeals ruling in 2003 that the DEA had overstepped its authority in listing hemp as a schedule I substances. The material is, therefore, still legal to grow and sell in the United States, provided that its THC level is below that specified for marijuana products.

HIA achieved another important breakthrough in 2010 when it purchased the diaries of Lyster Dewey, a project once again financed by Dr. Bronner's Magic Soap. (David Bronner, current president of Bronner's Magic Soaps, is past president of HIA and a current member of the organization's board of advisors.) Lyster Dewey has been described by hemp authority David P. West as "unarguably the most significant individual in US hemp history." West makes that assessment because of Dewey's role in the study of hemp at the U.S. Department of Agriculture (USDA) from 1890 to 1935. Dewey joined the department as "assistant to the botanist" in 1890 and remained with the department for all but the last two years of his life. In 1912, he began a hemp breeding program that by 1917, was beginning to produce healthier, more productive varieties of the cannabis plant. The interesting point that connects Dewey with HIA was the discovery of Dewey's notebooks at a yard sale in Amherst, New York, in 2010. The notebooks not only tell about Dewey's work with the cannabis plant, but provide photograph evidence of the success of his research. Perhaps most interesting of all, at least from a public relations standpoint, was the discovery that Dewey conducted much of his cannabis research on the present site of the Pentagon, the home of the U.S. military. HIA took advantage of this discovery by announcing the First Annual Hemp History Week in May 2010, celebrating, among other things, the discovery of Dewey's notebooks. Reports of that event told of nearly 200 events in 32 states, including programs in support of House Bill 1866, the Industrial Hemp Farming Act of 2009, introduced by Representative Ron Paul (R-TX).

Among its activities, the HIA has developed (in conjunction with Vote Hemp) Test Pledge, a voluntary testing program through which hemp growers pledge that the level of THC contained within their products is less than can be detected by any marijuana test. The association has also developed standards for hemp fibers indicating whether such fibers are pure hemp (Pure Hemp), more than half hemp but less than 100 percent (Hemp Rich), or more than 20 percent hemp but less than 50 percent (Hemp Content). The HIA website also has a rich resources section that lists many books, periodicals, reports, scientific studies, websites, and other resources of information about hemp.

John W. Huffman (1932–)

Huffman is best known for having developed a group of synthetic compounds that produce physiological effects similar to those caused by Δ^9-tetrahydrocannabinol (THC), the principal psychoactive component of marijuana. These synthetic cannabinoids are chemical analogs of THC, that is, they have the same basic structure as THC but differ in groups that have been substituted on the basic molecule. The compounds are known by abbreviations such as JWH-007, JWH-081, and JWH-398, where the "JWH" part of the name are Huffman's own initials. Huffman spent a significant portion of his academic career working on the development of these compounds, which are used primarily for two research purposes. First, they can be used to obtain additional information about cannabinoid receptors in the endocannabinoid system. Scientists now know that cannabinoids produce their psychoactive effects by attaching to receptor sites in the brain and peripheral nervous system, setting off a chain of chemical reactions. What they know little about is the chemical structure of those receptors. The chemical structure of Huffman's synthetic cannabinoids can be used to solve that problem by finding out which compounds (and therefore which structures) activate receptor sites, thereby elucidating the three-dimensional structure of the receptor sites. The second purpose of the research, arising out of these discoveries, is the development of new pharmaceuticals that can produce cannabis-like physical effects such as increasing one's appetite, reducing nausea, and treating glaucoma.

Huffman's research has been enormously useful in providing researchers with a better understanding of the way the endocannabinoid system works. But that research has also gained a level of notoriety among the general public because of its use in developing new types of psychoactive drugs used for recreational purposes. These drugs are incorrectly known as *synthetic cannabis* when, in fact, they often consist of a mixture of traditional herbs with mild mood-altering properties (such as *Canavalia maritima, Nymphaea caerulea*, and *Scutellaria nana*) coated with one or more of Huffman's synthetic cannabinoids. The resulting product may have psychoactive effects more than a hundred times greater than that of THC. They are sold under a variety of names, including Spice, K2, Chronic Spice, Spice Gold, Spice Silver, Stinger, Yucatan Fire, Skunk, Pulse, and Black Mamba. When they first became available to the general public, they were legal because they contained no THC or other banned substance. Over time, however, a number of states in the United States and countries around the world have banned products of this kind.

Huffman himself has spoken out strongly about the risks involved in using synthetic cannabinoids as recreational drugs. The compounds were prepared, he points out, for research purpose, and little is known about their general effects on the body. Indeed, public health officials have reported emergency room visits as a result of using Spice, K2, and its analogs, a fact responsible for most of the bans now being adopted. The problem is that most of the now-illegal compounds are still generally available on the Internet.

John William Huffman was born in Evanston, Illinois, on July 21, 1932. He attended Northwestern University, which granted his BS in chemistry in 1954. He then continued his studies at Harvard University, where he earned his AM and his PhD in chemistry in 1956 and 1957, respectively. At Harvard, he studied under probably the century's greatest synthetic organic chemist, Robert B. Woodward. Huffman's first job was as assistant professor of chemistry at the Georgia Institute of Technology. He left Georgia Tech in 1960 to take a position at Clemson University as assistant professor of chemistry. Over time, he rose to the position of associate professor and then, in 1967, full professor at Clemson. He remained at Clemson until his retirement in 2005. He then continued to work at the university as research professor until he took full retirement in 2011. He also spent a year as visiting professor of chemistry at Colorado State University in 1982. During his career, Huffman published more than 100 papers in peer-reviewed journals.

Among the honors and awards granted Huffman have been NIH Career Development Award for 1965–1970, a Senior Scientist Award from the National Institute on Drug Abuse, a Clemson University Alumni Association Award for Outstanding Research Accomplishments, and a Raphael Mechoulam Annual Award in Cannabinoid Research.

In June 2011, Huffman talked with ABC News about the dangers of synthetic cannabinoids as recreational drugs. It would make more sense, he said, to legalize the use of marijuana, which has been thoroughly studied and whose effects are now well known. "The scientific evidence is," he explained, "that it's not a particularly dangerous drug," and, in any case, it is much less dangerous than the poorly understood and potentially highly risky synthetic cannabinoids.

International Association for Cannabinoid Medicines
Am Mildenweg 6
59602 Ruethen
Germany
Phone: +49-2952-9708571
Fax: +49-2952-902651
E-mail: info@cannabis-med.org
URL: http://www.cannabis-med.org/

The International Association for Cannabinoid Medicines (IACM) was founded in March 2000 for the purpose of advancing knowledge about cannabis, cannabinoids, and the endocannabinoid system and related topics. (The endocannabinoid system is a collection of fatty acid derivatives that occur in animal bodies and the receptor sites to which they bond. The endocannabinoid system is implicated in a number of fundamental physiological responses such as appetite, pain sensation, mood, and memory.) A major mission of the organization is to discover and distribute information related to how information about cannabinoids can be used for therapeutic purposes. In 2009, the organization changed its original name, International Association for Cannabis as Medicine to its current name. The change in name reflected a recognition by the organization that research has found a number of substances that affect cannabinoid receptors beyond cannabis itself and that a wider range of researchers should be attracted to the services that the association offers. The IACM statement of mission identifies five primary areas of concern:

• Support for research on cannabinoid products and the endocannabinoid system
• Promotion of the exchange of information about cannabinoids and the endocannabinoid system among researchers, health care practitioners, patients, and the general public
• Preparation and distribution of information about the pharmacology, toxicology, and therapeutic applications of cannabinoids and modulators of the endocannabinoid system

- Monitoring international and national developments related to therapeutic applications of the cannabinoids

- Cooperation with other organizations whose goals and mission are similar to those of the International Association for Cannabinoid Medicine.

The three most important functions of the association are its website, its two major publications, and its annual conference. The IACM website is a treasure trove of information on the medicine, science, and law related to cannabinoids and the endocannabinoid system. For example, the section on medicine includes reports on medical uses of the cannabinoids, reported side effects of the use of cannabinoids, and a large selection of studies and case reports. The section on science provides definitions of important terms used in discussing cannabinoids and the endocannabinoid system, a list of clinical studies with descriptions of their general findings, an interactive database of clinical studies, and a comprehensive review and commentary of studies on cannabinoids and the endocannabinoid system between 2005 and 2009. The law and politics section provides a general summary of the legal status of cannabinoid therapeutics in about a dozen countries, including Canada, Finland, France, Germany, Israel, New Zealand, Spain, Sweden, the Netherlands, the United Kingdom, and the United States. Each of these summaries discusses laws dealing with the therapeutic uses of cannabinoids, court rulings, and a review of the legal and political "realities" in each country.

IACM makes available two essential publications in the field of cannabinoid therapeutics. One is the *Cannabinoids*, a peer-reviewed journal published electronically on an irregular, as-needed basis. It consists of mini-reviews of recent medical and scientific research, ideas, and issues; commentaries on other articles in the field of cannabinoid therapeutics; and letters about relevant topics in the field. Another publication of IACM was the short-lived *Journal of Cannabis Therapeutics*, which produced 10 issues between 2001 and 2004, at which time it discontinued publication. *IACM Bulletin* is a free, biweekly, online publication that covers every aspect of cannabinoid therapeutics. The December 18, 2011 issue, for example, contained an article about Roger Pertwee, long-term board member of IACM and winner of the 2011 Wellcome Gold Medal; a report of research on the effect of cannabis on blood levels of appetite hormones of individuals with HIV/AIDS; and a summary of "news in brief" about recent research and legalization activities. All past copies of the *IACM Bulletin* are available in the archives section of the organization's website.

The IACM's other major activity is a biannual conference, held in odd-numbered years at various locations. The 2011 conference was held on September 8 through 10 in Bonn, Germany. Previous conferences were held in Berlin (2001), Cologne (2003, 2007, and 2009), and Leiden (2005).

The IACM also contains a frequently asked questions (FAQ) section that provides answers to fundamental questions about cannabinoid therapeutics on topics such as anxiety, gastric ulcers, cognitive performance, risks of smoking cannabis, chromosomal damage, male fertility, asthma, and pregnancy.

R. Gil Kerlikowske (1949–)

Kerlikowske is the sixth director of the White House Office of National Drug Control Policy (ONDCP). He was appointed to that position by President Barack Obama and, after confirmation by the U.S. Senate, took office on May 7, 2009. He has been described by one independent website (NNDB; http://www.nndb.com/people/547/000204932/) as "less than an absolute absolutist on recreational drugs." That opinion is based to some extent on Kerlikowske's position on the issue while chief of the Seattle (Washington) Police Department, where he said that arresting individuals for simple marijuana possession was "not a priority." He focused on directing marijuana users into treatment programs rather than pushing for their incarceration. In spite of this perception, Kerlikowske has spoken almost as harshly about the legal status of marijuana as have all of his predecessors. At a press conference in Fresno, California, in 2009, following a $1.2 billion marijuana raid, he was quoted as saying that "[l]egalization is not in the president's vocabulary, and it's not in mine. Marijuana is dangerous and has no medicinal benefit."

Richard Gil Kerlikowske was born on November 23, 1949, in Fort Meyers, Florida, to Norma Shands, whom he acknowledged during his confirmation hearings for her strong support while he was growing up. Kerlikowske's stepfather was Judge Thomas W. Shands, whom he also praised during those hearings. Kerlikowske attended Fort Meyers High School, from which he graduated in 1968. He joined the U.S. Army in 1970, where he was assigned to the military police. Upon his discharge, Kerlikowske joined the St. Petersburg (Florida) Police Department, where he served with distinction until 1985. During his tenure in St. Petersburg, Kerlikowske also pursued a college education, earning his BA and MA, both in criminal justice, from the University of South Florida at Tampa in 1975 and 1978, respectively. In 1984, he also completed studies at the National Executive Institute of the Federal Bureau of Investigations Academy in Quantico, Virginia.

In 1987, Kerlikowske accepted an appointment as chief of the Port St. Lucie (Florida) Police Department, where he served until 1990. He then moved to a similar position with the Fort Pierce (Florida) Police Department. In 1994, he took a new job as police commissioner for the city of Buffalo, New York, where he remained until 1998. In that year, he became deputy director of the U.S. Department of Justice Office of Community Oriented Policing Services. After spending two years at that post, Kerlikowske was appointed chief of the Seattle Police Department, a post he held until President Obama nominated him to become director of the White House ONDCP.

In addition to his work in law enforcement, Kerlikowske has been active in professional and advocacy organizations. He has served as chair of the board of directors of Fight Crime: Invest in Kids, a national organization that works to prevent children and adolescents from becoming involved in crime. He served twice as president of the Major Cities Chiefs, an organization consisting of the largest law enforcement agencies in the United States and Canada. He was also a member of board of directors of the Salvation Army in both Buffalo and Seattle.

The first of Kerlikowske's many honors was the Presidential Service Badge, awarded him while he served in the military police. He has also received the Gary Hayes National Memorial Award for Innovation in Policing of the Police Executive Research Forum in 1990, and the organization's Leadership Award in 2006, and the American Medical Association's Dr. Nathan Davis Award for Outstanding Government Service in 2011. In 2010, his alma mater, the University of South Florida, awarded him an honorary Doctorate in Humane Letters degree in recognition of his contribution to law enforcement.

Marijuana Policy Project
236 Massachusetts Ave. NE, Suite 400
Washington, DC 20002
Phone: (202) 462-5747
URL: http://www.mpp.org/
Email: info@mpp.org

The Marijuana Policy Project (MPP) was founded in 1995 by Rob Kampia, Chuck Thomas, and Mike Kirshner, former members of the National Organization for the Reform of Marijuana Laws (NORML), after an internal disagreement about proposed changes in the parent organization. MPP was chartered in the District of Columbia as a nonprofit association lobbying for changes in the legal status of marijuana. The organization continues as a lobbying organization, while also maintaining a 501(c)(4) tax-free educational foundation, the MPP Foundation, to which charitable contributions can be made. MPP's mission statement consists of four major objectives: "(1) increase public support for non-punitive, non-coercive marijuana policies; (2) identify and activate supporters of non-punitive, non-coercive marijuana policies; (3) change state laws to reduce or eliminate penalties for the medical and non-medical use of marijuana; and (4) gain influence in Congress." Its corresponding vision statement calls for a nation in which marijuana is regulated in much the same way that alcohol currently is, in which education about marijuana use is "honest and realistic," and in which treatment for those who abuse marijuana is provided in a noncoercive way aimed at reduced harm to the individual.

The work of the Marijuana Policy Project is divided into a half-dozen major areas. In the field of legislation, it promotes the filing, consideration, and adoption of laws at the federal and state level designed to reduce harsh legal penalties for the use of marijuana. It has also developed a model state medical marijuana law for legislators' consideration. MPP also works at both federal and state levels to influence legislative action on all phases of marijuana laws, including medical marijuana policies and laws in particular. The Marijuana Policy Project also organizes and conducts a number of marijuana-related campaigns that deal with a changing set of themes such as (in 2012) the California Voter Education Project, the Marijuana Policy Project of California, the Massachusetts Patient Advocacy Alliance, the War on Drug Czar, the Nationwide Radio Ads program, the Mandatory Madness campaign against mandatory sentencing for marijuana convictions, and a campaign for legalizing and taxing marijuana.

Another area of focus for MPP is its Patients campaign, which collects and distributes stories of specific individuals who require and/or have used marijuana for medical purposes. The organization's website carries these stories on its Patients page. Finally, the organization's Victims campaign tells the stories of individuals who have become enmeshed in the legal system because of their possession and/or use of marijuana.

MPP also organizes its work into a number of issues areas that deal with specific aspects of the marijuana legalization effort. In 2012, those issues included collateral sanctions, courts and the justice system, drug testing and employment, enforcement and policing, the marijuana market and the economy, medical marijuana, the ONDCP and the drug czar, scientific studies and research, search and seizure, and teenagers and the gateway theory.

The Marijuana Policy Project is a rich source of written and electronic articles and reports on many aspects of the legalization of marijuana. They include items such as PDF files on "Know the Facts," "Marijuana Prohibition Facts," "Marijuana Policy Map," "Tax & Regulate: Effective Arguments," "Top Ten Reasons to Tax & Regulate Marijuana," "Dollars and Common Sense: Summary and Arguments for MPP's Decriminalization Bill," "MPP's Model Decriminalization Bill," "State Polling," "Federal Obstruction of Medical Marijuana Research Memo," and "Federal Enforcement Policy De-Prioritizing Medical Marijuana." Other articles and reports available from MPP include "Overview and Explanation of MPP's Model State Medical Marijuana Bill," "Marijuana and DUI Laws: How Can We Best Guard against Impaired Driving?" "Marijuana: Myths vs. Reality," "Implications of U.S. Supreme Court Medical Marijuana Ruling," "Common Questions about Marijuana," "Treatment for Marijuana Problems: Separating Fact from Fiction," "Medical Marijuana Overview," "Model State Medical Marijuana Bill," and "Questions and Answers About SATIVEX Liquid Medical Marijuana."

The Marijuana Policy Project claims to be the largest organization in the United States working solely on the issue of legalization of marijuana, with more than 32,000 members in all 50 states, the District of Columbia, Puerto Rico, Canada, Great Britain, Australia, and other international locations.

Raphael Mechoulam (1930–)

Mechoulam is professor of medicinal chemistry and natural products at the Hebrew University of Jerusalem, Israel. He is best known for having isolated, determined the chemical structure of, and synthesized Δ^9-tetrahydrocannabinol, best known as THC, the primary psychoactive ingredient in cannabis.

Raphael Mechoulam was born in Sofia, Bulgaria, on November 5, 1930. His father was a physician and head of a local hospital. His mother was not employed, but, as he later told an interviewer with the Endocannabinoid System Network (ESN), "enjoyed the life of a well-to-do Jewish family." Mechoulam attended the American Grade School in Sofia, "the only regular schooling" he could remember, as he told the ESN interviewer. As World War II approached, life for the Mechoulams became much more difficult because of the anti-Semitic laws adopted by the Nazi-leaning Bulgarian government. The family was forced to move from village to village seeking enough work to survive. Eventually, Raphael's father was sent to a concentration camp, an experience he survived. Mechoulam was able to obtain only one year of secondary education, at Sofia's First Male Gymnasium, where he had his first exposure to chemical engineering, an experience that he later said he did not enjoy.

As circumstances in Bulgaria became ever more difficult for Jewish families, the Mechoulams finally decided to emigrate to Israel in 1949. There Raphael enrolled at the Hebrew University at Jerusalem, from which he received his MSc in biochemistry in 1952. It was not until he began his military service a year later, however, that he really became interested in scientific research. His assignment in the military involved a research project on insecticides. It was as a result of that experience, he later told an ESN interviewer, that he "found the independence of research to be an addiction from which I do not want to be cured."

Upon completing his military service in 1956, Mechoulam designed to return to academia, beginning his doctoral studies at the Weizmann Institute in Rehovot, Israel. He completed his studies and was granted his PhD in steroid studies in 1958. After a two-year postdoctoral program at the Rockefeller Institute in New York, Mechoulam returned to Israel, where he served first as junior scientist, and later as senior scientist, at the Weizmann Institute from 1960 to 1965. His research assignments at Weizmann involved the study of natural products such as alkaloids, terpenes, and cannabinoids. It was during his tenure at Weizmann that Mechoulam and his colleagues first identified THC as the primary psychoactive compound in cannabis and then were able to synthesize the substance in the laboratory. The accomplishment was significant because cannabis was at the time one of the most poorly understood of all psychoactive compounds. Laws against its possession made research difficult and without access to the pure substance, learning more about its chemical structure and properties were difficult. Mechoulam's research changed that scenario and made it possible for researchers to mount an aggressive campaign to understand more about the compound and the mechanisms by which it acts in animal bodies.

Mechoulam's discoveries about THC marked only the beginning of a lifelong study of the whole cannabinoid family. He eventually isolated and identified a large number of naturally occurring members of the family. In 1992, Mechoulam's research took a somewhat different direction when his research team identified the first endocannabinoid, which they named anandamide (which means "bliss" in Sanskrit). Endocannabinoids are substances produced by animal bodies that activate cannabinoid receptors in the body and, thus, have psychoactive effects similar to those of natural cannabinoids like THC. In 1995, Mechoulam's research team discovered a second endocannabinoid, arachidonoyl glycerol (2- AG), which occurs in the intestines. Today, Mechoulam remains a major figure in research on cannabinoids and endocannabinoids.

In 1966, Mechoulam accepted an appointment at Hebrew University, where he was later promoted to associate professor in 1968 and full professor in 1972. In 1975, he was named Lionel Jacobson Professor of Medicinal Chemistry, a post he continues to hold. From 1979 to 1982, he was named rector (academic head) of Hebrew University; from 1983 to 1985, he served as prorector (an officer who presides over the academic senate of a German univeristy) of the university. From 1993 to 1994, Mechoulam was also visiting professor in the Department of Pharmacology at the Medical College of Richmond, in Richmond, Virginia.

During his career, Mechoulam has received a number of honors and awards, including the Somach Sachs Prize for the best research by a scientist under the age of 35 at the Weizmann Institute (1964); the Kolthof Prize in Chemistry from The Technion, Haifa, Israel (1994); election as a member of the Israel Academy of Sciences (1994); the Hanus Medal of the Czech Chemical Society (1998); the David R. Bloom Prize of the Center for Pharmacy at Hebrew University (1998); the Israel Prize in Exact Sciences (2000); the Heinrich Wieland Prize, endowed by Boehringer-Ingelheim (2004); the Henrietta Szold Prize for achievements in medical research, awarded by the city of Tel-Aviv (2005); the Lifetime Achievement Award of the European College of Neuropsychopharmacology (2006); a Special Award of the International Association for Cannabinoids in Medicine (2007); the Israel Chemical Society Prize for Excellence in Research (2009); Lifetime Achievement Awards from Hebrew University (2010) and the Eicosanoid Research Society (2011); and the NIDA [National Institute on Drug Abuse] Discovery Award (2011). In 1999, in Mechoulam's honor, the International Cannabinoid Research Society established an annual award to be named The R. Mechoulam Annual Award in Cannabinoid Research. Mechoulam has also received honorary doctorates from Ohio State University and Complutense University, Madrid. In addition to numerous peer-reviewed scientific papers, Mechoulam has edited four books, has published numerous book chapters, and has been awarded 25 patents for his new discoveries.

Tod Hiro Mikuriya (1933–2007)

Mikuriya was possibly the best known medical professional working for the legalization of marijuana for medical purposes.

He first became interested in the topic during the 1960s, during which time he was briefly director of nonclassified marijuana research at the National Institute of Mental Health Center for Narcotics and Drug Abuse Studies (1967). He came to the conclusion that government officials and many medical researchers were largely ignoring a vast body of research on the medical benefits of marijuana and were focusing instead on any and all research reporting the harmful effects of the plant. In 1972, he self-published the book for which he is perhaps best known, *Marijuana Medical Papers, 1839–1972*. The book contained about two dozen papers dealing with the medical effects of marijuana, personal experiences with the drug, discussions of the therapeutic value of marijuana, recent clinical studies, chemical and pharmacological research, and a social history of the origin of marijuana laws. Among the papers included in the book are an early (1839) scientific paper on the medical effects of marijuana by W. B. O'Shaughnessy, a report on the medical effects of *Cannabis indica* by the Ohio State Medical Committee on Cannabis Indica in 1860, a review of the La Guardia Committee report on marijuana of 1944, a section from the *Dispensatory of the United States* for 1918 that contains a description of the medical uses of marijuana, a paper on the relative effects of alcohol and marijuana on driving ability (1969), and an analysis of the 1937 Marihuana Tax Act as a commentary on the social origins of marijuana laws.

Tod Hiro Mikuriya was born on September 20, 1933, in Bucks County, Pennsylvania, to Tadafumi Mikuriya, a former Japanese samurai who had converted to Christianity and became a civil engineer who specialized in bridge design, and Anna Schwenk Mikuriya, a German immigrant who taught special education. Tod received his secondary education at George School in Newtown, Pennsylvania (1948–1951), and then matriculated at Haverford College, in Haverford, Pennsylvania, both Quaker institutions. In 1954, Mikuriya was expelled from Haverford for allegedly being involved in panty raids at nearby Bryn Mawr College (an act to which he later admitted his guilt), and he transferred to yet another Quaker institution, Guilford College in Greensboro, North Carolina. He remained at Guilford for only one semester before changing institutions once more, this time to Reed College, in Portland, Oregon, from which he finally received his bachelor's degree in psychology in 1956. He is reported to have earned his way through college by writing and singing folk songs, an interest he retained throughout his life. After graduating from Reed, Mikuriya was drafted into the U.S. Army, where he served as a neuropsychiatric technician until he was discharged in 1958. He then continued his studies at Temple University, from which he received his MD in 1962. He later reported that his lifelong interest in marijuana was triggered by an article about the medical uses of marijuana that he read at Temple. Mikuriya completed his internship at Southern Pacific Hospital (later Harkness Community Hospital and now closed) and his psychiatric residencies at the Oregon State Hospital, in Salem, and the Mendocino State Hospital, in Talmage, California.

In October 1966, Mikuriya was appointed director of the Drug Addiction Treatment Center at the New Jersey NeuroPsychiatric Institute in Princeton, New Jersey, a post he held for 10 months. He then accepted a job as director of marijuana research at the Center for Narcotics and Drug Abuse Studies of the National Institute of Mental Health. He left that post after only three months because he had become convinced that his superiors were interested only in marijuana research with negative connotations. Mikuriya then moved to the West Coast, where he served as consulting psychiatrist at the Alameda County Alcoholism Clinic and the county Health Department Drug Abuse Program in 1968 and 1969. In 1970, he went into private practice in Berkeley while also acting as attending staff psychiatrist at the Gladman Hospital in Oakland, California. He remained active until a few weeks before his death on May 20, 2007, in Berkeley.

In addition to his private practice, Mikuriya was active in organizations that were interested in the use of marijuana for medical purposes, as well as a number of professional organizations, including the Drug Use and Abuse Committee of the Northern California Psychiatric Society, the National Commission on Marihuana and Drug Abuse, the Biofeedback Society of California, and the Society of Cannabis Clinicians, of which he was founder. For a major part of his life, Mikuriya was essentially the only physician who advocated publicly and enthusiastically for the use of marijuana to treat a variety of medical conditions. In 1996, he helped draft California Proposition 215, which legalized the use of marijuana for medical conditions.

As part of the campaign in support of Proposition 215, Mikuriya distributed a list of medical conditions for which marijuana could be used in treatment, a list compiled from the historic medical literature. After the proposition passed, U.S. Drug Czar Barry McCaffrey held a press conference threatening to prosecute any California doctor who wrote prescriptions for marijuana under the recently adopted California law. At that conference, where he was joined by Secretary of Heath, Education, and Welfare Donna Shalala and Alan Lesher of the National Institute on Drug Abuse, McCaffrey said of Mikuriya's list of medical conditions, "This isn't medicine. This is a Cheech and Chong Show." (Cheech and Chong were two stand-up comedians from the 1970s and 1980s who supposedly typified the strange behavior of marijuana-addicted hippies.)

In 2000, the California Medical Board investigated Mikuriya for using marijuana in the treatment of some of his patients. The complaint was brought not by the patients, but by law enforcement officers. The board fined him $75,000 and placed him on probation, but he continued to practice under supervision. He announced that he would continue to appeal the board's decision, and did follow that path until his health made it impossible for him to pursue the issue further. Mikuriya had announced plan for an updated and expanded version of *Marijuana Medical Papers*, a project he was unable to complete before his death.

National Institute on Drug Abuse

National Institutes of Health
6001 Executive Blvd., Room 5213
Bethesda, MD 20892-9561
Phone: (301) 443-1124
E-mail: information@nida.nih.gov
URL: http://www.nida.nih.gov/nidahome.html

The origins of the federal government's interest in drug abuse issues can be traced to 1935 with the establishment of a research facility at the U.S. Public Health Service (USPHS) hospital in Lexington, Kentucky. Originally called the U.S. Narcotics Farm, the facility was a joint project of the USPHA and the U.S. Bureau of Prisons. It eventually underwent a number of name changes. In 1948, the facility because the Addiction Research Center and in 1967, the National Institute of Mental Health Clinical Research Center. The National Institute on Drug Abuse (NIDA) was created in 1972 by Public Law 92-255, the Drug Abuse Office and Treatment Act of 1972, to become operational in 1974 as a division within the National Institute of Mental Health (NIMH). NIDA's mission was to be responsible for developing a national community-based treatment system and a program for treatment of narcotic addicts. A year later, a reorganization act created the Alcohol, Drug Abuse, and Mental Health Administration (ADAMHA), an umbrella organization of NIDA, NIMH, and the National Institute on Alcohol Abuse and Alcoholism. In 1992, another reorganization act moved the NIDA from ADAMHA to the National Institutes of Health, where it resides today.

The primary responsibility of the NIDA is to sponsor and conduct research on all aspects of substance use and abuse. This charge includes research on topics such as the genetic, neurobiological, behavioral, and social mechanisms underlying drug abuse and addiction; the causes and consequences of substance abuse, including issues of concern to special populations such as ethnic minorities, youth, and women; the relationship of substance abuse to other forms of mental illness and to related issues such as unemployment, low socioeconomic status, and violence; effective methods of prevention and treatment, including new medications and behavioral therapies for drug addiction; the relationship of substance abuse to cultural and ethical issues such as health disparities; and the relationship of substance abuse to the acquisition, transmission, and clinical course of diseases such as HIV/AIDS, tuberculosis, and other diseases.

NIDA's work is carried out through nine divisions and offices concerned with specific aspects of the organization's mission. For example, the Division of Epidemiology, Services, and Prevention Research is responsible for a broad extramural research program on topics such as the nature, patterns, and consequences of drug use among general, special, and community-based populations; prevention of substance abuse and addiction; behavioral and social science research among communities and specialized populations; and economic modeling and structuring of treatment systems. The Division of Basic Neuroscience and Behavioral Research focuses on studies of the neurobiological and behavioral actions of legal and illegal drugs. The Division of Clinical Neuroscience and Behavioral Research deals with applications of neurobiological research to real-life substance abuse issues. The Division of Pharmacotherapies and Medical Consequences of Drug Abuse is responsible for the design, development, FDA approval and marketing of new medications for the treatment of drug-related disorders and addictions.

One of NIDA's signature programs is its Monitoring the Future survey, conducted annually since 1975. The survey is designed to provide an overview of drugs use by high school students and their attitudes toward drug abuse. Originally aimed at twelfth graders throughout the United States, in 1991, the survey was extended to include eighth and tenth graders. Another important NIDA function, its Research Monographs Series, was also initiated in 1975. The series is designed to make available to specialists in the field the most recent information about scientific research on substance abuse and related issues. A third important NIDA program, the Drug Abuse Information and Treatment Referral Hotline, was initiated in 1986 and continues to be an essential feature of the agency's services.

NIDA produces a large range of print and electronic media for specialists in the field of substance abuse, for the medical profession in general, for parents, and for students. These publications cover all types of illegal and legal abused substances such as cocaine, heroin, nicotine, prescription medications, and anabolic steroids. Some examples of the materials about marijuana include "Marijuana: Facts for Teens" (English and Spanish); "Marijuana: Facts Parents Need to Know" (English and Spanish); "Mind over Matter: The Brain's Response to Marijuana"; and "NIDA Research Report Series: Marijuana." The agency also provides serial publications, including *NIDA Notes*, a (usually) biannual publication of research and other news related to substance abuse; *NIDA InfoFacts*, a series of publications on specific topics in substance abuse such as drugged driving, comorbidity, khat (a plant whose leaves are chewed for their stimulant effects primarily in East Africa and the Arabian peninsula), and inhalants; *NIDA Addiction Science & Clinical Practice*, a biannual journal of scientific developments in the field of substance abuse; and *Topics in Brief*, occasional publications dealing with topics of current interest in substance abuse such as smokeless tobacco, medications development at NIDA, and prenatal exposure to drugs of abuse. Among the agency's most useful resources for the general public is its set of fact sheets on a variety of drugs and related topics. The current series includes fact sheets on drugs ranging from alcohol and club drugs to methamphetamine and phencyclidine, as well as topics that include addiction science, clinical trials networks, drug use and mental illness, drug testing, prevention research, treatment research, and trends and statistics.

NIDA also sponsors conferences and other meetings throughout the year on substance abuse issues. Meetings held in

November 2011, for example, dealt with the science of abuse liability assessment, frontiers in addiction research, and a NIDA/NIH grant workshop for early career researchers.

National Organization for the Reform of Marijuana Laws (dba NORML)

1600 K St., NW, Mezzanine Level
Washington, DC 20006-2832
Phone: (202) 483-5500
Fax: (202) 483-0057
E-mail: norml@norml.org
URL: http://norml.org/

NORML was founded in 1970 by attorney Keith Stroup with a $5,000 grant from the Playboy Foundation. According to NORML's Policy on Personal Use, the organization "supports the removal of all penalties for the private possession of marijuana by adults, cultivation for personal use, and the casual nonprofit transfers of small amounts. NORML also supports the development of a legally controlled market for marijuana." Although NORML is not a tax-deductible organization, its sister association, the NORML Foundation is a 501(c)(3) tax-deductible organization. The NORML Foundation was established in 1997 with the goal of informing and educating the American public about the costs associated with prohibiting marijuana use and the benefits of pursuing alternative policies. The foundation also provides legal support and assistance to individuals who have been or are being persecuted under existing laws.

NORML has its main headquarters in Washington, DC, with 108 state chapters in every state of the union, plus international chapters in Brazil, Norway, Spain, South Africa, Australia, and New Zealand (five chapters). Depending on the geographic region served, chapters are designated as regional chapters, chapters, or subchapters.

NORML's work focuses on four major areas: research on marijuana use, the use of marijuana for medical purposes, legal assistance for individuals arrested for marijuana-related crimes, and public education. In the area of research, the organization has been collecting information on the personal, medical, and industrial uses of cannabis products for more than 40 years. A collection of that information is now available on the organization's website at http://norml.org/library. The website also contains detailed information about laws dealing with marijuana production, transport, and use. The area of the site for doctors and patients deals with all aspects of the medical marijuana issue, including a general overview of the topic, reports on the use of marijuana for medical purposes, health reports, and a detailed review of the legal availability of medical marijuana in various parts of the country. A guide to marijuana dispensaries is also available on the website through an external source at http://legalmarijuanadispensary.com/.

The organization's Legal page provides a list of lawyers with special interest and expertise in the field of marijuana issues, including the field of medical marijuana. It also has a Legal Brief Bank page with special resources on topics such as constitutional challenges to marijuana laws, medical marijuana issues, search and seizure, challenges to marijuana laws based on religious arguments, state laws on marijuana, drug testing, drug scheduling laws and regulations, and a variety of miscellaneous issues. NORML's page on Busted? provides practical information for individuals who have been arrested for a marijuana-related crime. In addition to providing suggestions for attorneys and legal defenses, the page suggests immediate actions one can take in response to a recent arrest. Historical data on arrests are also provided.

Another section of the organization's website deals with drug testing issues, including a general overview of the philosophy behind drug testing and the methodologies used in the procedure. It also provides detailed information about the process involved in carrying out a drug test, along with advice for individuals who may be required to undergo drug testing for marijuana.

One of the most useful services provided by NORML is an extended and detailed online library with separate sections on economic reports, driving and marijuana, reports on legalization, European drug laws, health reports, reports on the production and use of hemp, marijuana crop reports, comparisons of natural and synthetic marijuana, medical marijuana reports, requests for information under the U.S. Freedom of Information Act, surveys and polls, and public testimony about the legalization of marijuana. Two of NORML's major online publications are the *NORML Big Book of Facts* and the 2005 publication *Truth Report 2005, Your Government Is Lying to You (Again) about Marijuana*.

An additional major component of NORML's work is an annual conference as well as various state and regional conferences. The first NORML conference, the People's First Pot Conference, was held in Washington, DC, in 1972. It has been repeated every year since. Video and written records of many of those conferences are available on the NORML website at http://norml.org/component/zoo/category/norml-conferences. The 2011 conference included sessions on topics such as "Pot-n-Politics: 2011-2012 Marijuana Initiatives"; "Cannabis Commerce: Coming of Age"; "NORML Women's Alliance: Closing The Cannabis Gender Gap"; "Medical Marijuana: More Than Just THC"; "Medibles: Cannabis & Cooking"; "NORML at 40-Years-Old"; "Marijuana and Safety: Real Myths, Real Concerns"; "The Feds, Marijuana, and You"; and "Marijuana Nation: The Statistics of Cannabis and Its Consumers."

Office of National Drug Control Policy
The White House
1600 Pennsylvania Ave., NW
Washington, DC 20500
Phone: (202) 395-6618
E-mail: http://www.whitehouse.gov/ondcp/contact
URL: http://www.whitehouse.gov/ondcp

The Office of National Drug Control Policy (ONDCP) was established in 1989 as a provision of the Anti-Drug Abuse Act of 1988. Attached to the director's office are administrative units that include the offices of the Legal Counsel, Research and Data Analysis, Legislative Affairs, Management and Administration, Public Affairs, Performance and Budget, and Intergovernmental Public Liaison. The three programmatic offices attached to the director's office deal with demand reduction; supply reduction; and state, local, and tribal affairs. In its 2011 budget, ONDCP requested a staff of 98 full-time employees, of whom about two-thirds would be employed at pay grades of GS-14, GS-15, or SES with a minimum salary of $105,211 per year. The office's mission is to advise the president on drug-control issues, coordinate drug-control activities and related funding across the federal government, and produce the annual National Drug Control Strategy. This document outlines efforts by the federal government to reduce illicit drug use, manufacturing and trafficking, drug-related crime and violence, and drug-related health consequences.

Under the administration of President Barack Obama, ONDCP has taken a somewhat different approach to the nation's drug control problem than have earlier administrations. It is, according to its website, focusing on "renewed emphasis on community-based prevention programs, early intervention programs in healthcare settings, aligning criminal justice policies and public health systems to divert non-violent drug offenders into treatment instead of jail, funding scientific research on drug use, and, through the Affordable Care Act, expanding access to substance abuse treatment."

Much of the office's work is organized under one of about a half-dozen initiatives and key policies areas: prescription drug abuse, drugged driving, community-based drug prevention, healthcare, marijuana, methamphetamine, and public lands (where large quantities of cannabis are grown). The office takes among the strongest and most aggressive stands on the use of marijuana of any American organization. It warns that marijuana is "addictive and unsafe," especially for adolescents. Cannabis contains, the office warns, chemicals that "can change the way the brain works" and is associated with a host of mental and physical disorders, including "addiction, respiratory and mental illness, poor motor performance, and cognitive impairment." The office also campaigns strongly against the use of smoked marijuana for medicinal purposes. It acknowledges that although some orally administered components of cannabis may have medicinal value, "smoking marijuana is an inefficient and harmful method for delivering the constituent elements that have or may have medicinal value." It also reiterates the fact that while a number of states have legalized the use of marijuana for medicinal purposes, possession and use of the drug are illegal under federal law, and anyone who uses marijuana for medicinal purposes in any part of the nation is liable for arrest and prosecution under the Controlled Substances Act of 1970.

ONDCP has also developed programs for populations that it regards as being at special risk for drug abuse: military veterans and their families; women, children, and families; college and university students; and Native Americans and Alaska Natives. The office argues, for example, that men and women who have served in the military are at special risk for drug abuse both while they are in active service and after they have been discharged. They point to the high proportion of veterans who are currently serving prison terms and who are "struggling with substance abuse" (60 percent of 140,000 men and women). The office reminds members of the military and veterans of the host of services available for assistance with substance abuse such as the Substance Abuse Treatment Facility Locator of the Substance Abuse and Mental Health Services Administration (SAMHSA); the U.S. Department of Veterans Affairs; the National Association of Drug Court Professionals Veterans Treatment Courts Clearinghouse of the U.S. Department of Justice; the Veterans Suicide Prevention Hotline of SAMHSA;

the "Dealing With Effects of Trauma" self-help guide provided by SAMHSA; and the federal government's Veterans Employment Website of the Office of Personnel Management.

President Obama's emphasis on prevention and treatment is reflected in a number of well-developed programs for the general public in these two areas. The major focus of the ONDCP National Youth Anti-Drug Media Campaign, for example, is a program called Above the Influence, which includes both national-level advertising and targeted efforts at the local community level. A similar program is the ONDCP Drug-Free Communities Support Program, which provides federal grants to community-based coalitions working to prevent and reduce youth substance abuse. The other prong of President Obama's approach to substance abuse is treatment, with an emphasis on getting young substance abusers into treatment programs rather than prison systems. Existing federal and state services, as well as new programs, are available to achieve this objective.

The two primary components of supply reduction efforts by the office are international agreements and a strong enforcement program. The international programs involve agreements with Afghanistan, the Andean region, Canada, the Caribbean, Central America, Europe, Mexico, and Russia to reduce the production, processing, and distribution of illegal substances within and through these areas. The enforcement aspect of ONDCP's work focuses on the range of activities through which illegal substances are distributed in the United States. One of the major programs in this area is the High Intensity Drug Trafficking Area (HIDTA) Program, which targets regions where the transport and distribution of illegal substances is especially high.

ONDCP's most important publication is probably its *National Drug Control Strategy*, an annual publication that reviews the current status of substance abuse in the United States along with the federal government's plans for dealing with various aspects of that issue.

William B. O'Shaughnessy (1809–1889)

O'Shaughnessy was an Irish-born physician who introduced the use of cannabis products to Western medicine. Although he is probably best known for this accomplishment, he made other important contributions in a variety of fields, including laying the first telegraph system in Asia, developing a treatment for cholera, and inventing a system for laying telegraph systems under water.

William Brooke O'Shaughnessy was born in Limerick, Ireland, in 1809 to Daniel O'Shaughnessy and his wife (whose first name is not recorded, although her maiden name was Boswell). Little is known about his early life, but it is known that he was admitted to the University of Edinburgh in 1827, where he studied medicine, chemistry, anatomy, and forensic science. He received his medical degree from Edinburgh in 1829 but was unable to obtain a medical practice in London, where he had hoped to practice. Instead, he established his own forensic toxicology laboratory, where he carried out chemical analyses of blood, feces, urine, and tissue for doctors, hospitals, and the courts. In 1831, O'Shaughnessy made an important discovery concerning cholera. Cholera was (and still is) one of the most devastating of all diseases, in which death occurs because of persistent diarrhea and vomiting. O'Shaughnessy made what in retrospect appears to be a relatively simple suggestion, but one that had not yet been employed by the medical profession. Supplying a cholera victim with water and salts to replace those lost by vomiting and diarrhea, he said, could sustain their bodies and perhaps save their lives. In fact, when the practice was introduced in the treatment of cholera, up to half of all patients survived the disease.

In 1833, O'Shaughnessy accepted an appointment as assistant surgeon in the East India Company, with an assignment in Calcutta. His life in India was a busy one in which he not only served in his medical post, but also helped to found the Calcutta Medical College, where he also served as professor of chemistry and materia medica. He also became interested in the use of native materials for the treatment of diseases. In 1839, he read a 40-page paper on the subject to the Medical and Physical Society of Calcutta; this is sometimes said to be the first modern paper on the medical uses of cannabis. That paper is now considered a classic in the field of medicine, and certainly in the field of medical applications of cannabis. In the paper, O'Shaughnessy discusses the botanical and chemical characteristics of the plant, its popular uses, something of its known history, and six experiments he conducted to test its physical and medical effects on animals and humans. He concludes the paper with a review of the use of cannabis in the treatment of rheumatism, hydrophobia, cholera, infantile convulsions, and tetanus, the last of these perhaps the most influential portion of the paper for medical observers. In a short section at the end of the paper, he also reviews a type of delirium that results from overuse of the drug which, he says, is "easily treated."

During this period, O'Shaughnessy also became interested in the recently invented telegraph and pushed his military superiors to whom he was responsible for permission to construct a telegraph system in India. At the time, he received no encouragement from the governor general, Lord Ellenborough. Instead, exhausted by his many endeavors in the country, O'Shaughnessy requested and received a furlough that allowed him to return to England. During his visit home, he brought with him samples of cannabis used for medicinal purposes and began to write and speak about the potential applications of the drug. His work swept through the medical profession, and more than 100 scientific papers on the medical applications of cannabis were written between 1839 and 1900. In recognition of his work, Queen Victoria (who had taken cannabis for menstrual cramps) eventually knighted O'Shaughnessy (in 1856), and he was elected a member of the Royal Society in 1843.

In 1844, O'Shaughnessy returned to India and threw his energies into a new endeavor: working on a national telegraph system for India. By this time, a new governor general had been installed in India, Lord Dalhousie, who was much more receptive to O'Shaughnessy's plans for the telegraph. Dalhousie appointed O'Shaughnessy superintendent of telegraphy, and the cannabis proponent began work on the project. The challenges he faced were profound as he sought to lay down wires across inhospitable land using untrained laborers working with primitive equipment. Yet he was successful in his efforts, opening the first 27-mile segment of the system from Alipore to Diamond Harbor in 1852. At the time, the longest telegraph line in England was only two thirds as long, 18 miles. Eventually, O'Shaughnessy oversaw the completion of more than 4,000 lines of the telegraph system before he returned to England in 1855.

O'Shaughnessy's furlough in England was interrupted in 1857 when he returned once more to India in order to deal with the restoration and rebuilding of much of the telegraph system that had been destroyed during the Sepoy Mutiny of 1857. He ended his last tour of duty in India in 1861, when he retired from the East India Company and settled in the south of England. Almost nothing is known about the last 28 years of his life. He died in Southsea, England, on January 10, 1889.

Raymond P. Shafer (1917–2006)

Shafer was appointed in 1970 by President Richard M. Nixon to chair a commission studying the legal status of marijuana and drug abuse, the National Commission on Marihuana and Drug Abuse, a committee established by the U.S. Congress in October 1970. Nixon selected Shafer because he had a solid reputation as a strong antidrug person who was likely to produce a report that pointed out the harmful effects of marijuana and to call for severe restrictions on the drug's production, transport, and use. As it turned out, events did not develop in just that way as committee members from a wide variety of backgrounds—health experts, judges, probation officers, and clinicians—took seriously the charge of Public Law 91-513 and assembled an impressive collection of research, reports, and expert opinions on the topic. In the end, the commission produced a recommendation precisely the opposite of that expected by Nixon, calling for the legalization of marijuana. Whatever Shafer's own personal views on marijuana were, the commission's report ultimately represented the majority view of the best scientific information on the dangers (or lack of dangers) posed by legalization of marijuana.

Raymond Philip Shafer was born on March 5, 1917, in New Castle, Pennsylvania, to the Reverend David P. and Mina Belle Shafer. The family moved to Meadville, Pennsylvania, in 1933 when Rev. Shafer was offered a position at the First Christian Church there. Raymond graduated from Meadville High School in 1934, where he was valedictorian of his class and active in a variety of sports. He then matriculated at Allegheny College, where he served as class president for four years and president of the Allegheny Undergraduate Council. Shafer then went on to Yale Law School, where he was a member of an illustrious class that included future President Gerald Ford and Supreme Court Justices Potter Stewart and Byron White. He was granted his LLB by Yale in 1941. During World War II, Shafer served in Naval Intelligence and as captain of a PT (patrol torpedo) boat in the South Pacific. For his role in the war effort, he was awarded the Bronze Star and Purple Heart.

After the war, Shafer returned to Meadville, where he set up a law practice. In 1948, he made his first attempt at elected office and won the post of Crawford County District Attorney, a post in which he served until 1956. He then decided to run for statewide office and was elected senator from the Fiftieth District in 1958. He served in that post until 1962, beginning to establish himself as a moderate Republican on most issues. In March 1962, William M. Scranton, candidate for governor of the state, asked Shafer to join him on the ticket as candidate for lieutenant governor, an offer that Shafer accepted. The Scranton-Shafer ticket won the general election by almost 500,000 votes. Four years later, with Scranton prevented from serving a second term by the state constitution, Shafer became the Republican candidate for governor. He won that election also, this time by an even larger margin than in 1962. Shafer also served the one term permitted by the constitution, leaving office in 1971. Shafer's record as governor features his two special areas of interest: reform of the state constitution and development of the state's highway system, especially construction of the state's portion of the National System of Interstate and Defense Highways (the Interstate Highway System). Today, the portion of Interstate 79 that runs through Pennsylvania is known as the Raymond P. Shafer Highway.

After leaving the governor's office, Shafer remained active in the Republican Party, a stalwart member of its moderate wing. In 1968, he gave the presidential nominating speech at the Republican National Convention for Governor Nelson Rockefeller of New York, thereby earning the enmity of the eventual nominee, Richard Nixon. When searching for a chair of the marijuana commission, however, Nixon apparently overlooked his earlier concerns about Shafer, certain that the commission would produce the result that he wanted and anticipated. Which, as it turns out, was not the case.

After a brief foray into the private sector as chief executive officer (CEO) of the TelePrompter corporation, Shafer returned to federal service in 1974, when he served as special council to newly appointed Vice President Nelson Rockefeller. At the end of that tenure, he returned to private business permanently, serving as partner in the accounting firm of Coopers & Lybrand from 1977 to 1988. Shafer also served briefly as president of his alma mater, Allegheny College, from 1985 to 1986.

Shafer died in Meadville on December 12, 2006. In a somewhat ironic tribute to his work on marijuana, a 2011 bill dealing with medical marijuana use in Pennsylvania, House Bill 1652, was named The Governor Raymond P. Shafer Compassionate Use Medical Marijuana Act. The bill did not pass the legislature.

Keith Stroup (1943–)

Stroup is founder of the National Organization for the Reform of Marijuana Laws (NORML). He is an attorney and has spent most of his adult life on efforts to legalize the use of marijuana in the United States. He served as president of NORML from its founding in 1970 to 1979 and then returned to the organization as executive director from 1995 to 2004 and as legal counsel from 2005 to the present.

Keith Stroup was born in Dix, Illinois, on December 27, 1943. His parents were Russell Stroup, who had come from a farming family and was then a successful building contractor and unofficial head of the regional Republican Party, and Vera Stroup, whose father was a miner who died of black lung disease. Keith's childhood has been described by his biographer Patrick Anderson in his book *High in America: The True Story behind NORML and the Politics of Marijuana* "as American as apple pie." Keith and his older brother Larry were brought up in a strict Southern Baptist tradition in which all types of immoral behavior such as smoking, drinking, and dancing were prohibited. As the boys grew older, according to Anderson, Larry developed into a successful conservative businessman who married his high school sweetheart and remained loyal to the Pleasant Hill Baptist Church, while Keith began to rebel against the strictures of his parents' beliefs.

The turning point for Keith, according to Anderson, came when he entered high school in nearby Mount Vernon. Although he was successful academically and socially, Keith gradually grew further and further apart from his family. The final break seemed to come just after graduation when his parents angrily expelled a group of Keith's friends from the family home for playing poker and drinking beer. Outraged at this turn of events, Keith left for Yellowstone National Park without telling his family, returning to Illinois only to enter the University of Illinois in the fall of 1961. Only a short time into his college years at Illinois, he was expelled for violating university regulations at an off-campus party. The following year was one of uncertainty and confusion, spent as a furniture repossessor at a Portland (Oregon) loan company, a short-lived candidate for the Peace Corps, and a student for one term at a small college in Kentucky. He was finally readmitted to Illinois, from which he graduated with a BA in political science and sociology in 1965. He then continued his studies at the Georgetown University Law Center, from which he received his law degree in 1968. While at Georgetown, Stroup had a part-time job working for Senator Everett Dirkson (R-IL), earning $50 a week and gaining invaluable experience in the wheelings and dealings of Washington politics. Ironically, it is said that he got the job because of the influence of his father, who had remained a powerful voice in southern Illinois politics.

In the last few months before graduating from Georgetown, Stroup noticed an advertisement on a bulletin board for positions at the federal Consumer Product Safety Commission (CPSC). He applied for and received a job with the CPSC, where he came into contact with activist Ralph Nader. This experience provided Stroup with the opportunity to learn more about political activism and encouraged him to form a new organization devoted to the legalization of marijuana. Based on that background and with a grant of $5,000 from the Playboy Foundation, Stroup and a group of friends founded NORML in 1970. He continued to serve as executive director of the organization until 1979, when he was asked to leave by the organization's board of directors. The explanation for Stroup's removal from his post was that he had "outed" Dr. Peter Bourne, special advisor for health to President Jimmy Carter and de factor "drug czar" in the Carter administration, for using cocaine at a 1977 party they had both attended. Stroup, in turn, had been relieved of his NORML job apparently because the board of directors did not approve of "snitches" in its organization. Many years later, Stroup was to tell a *Washington Post* reporter that this episode was "probably the stupidest thing I ever did." By involving Bourne in a drug-related incident (which Bourne has always denied), Stroup lost a valuable contact with an administration that was, in fact, open to the possibility of changing federal regulations concerned with marijuana possession.

In any case, Stroup then cofounded his own law firm, Stroup, Goldstein, Jacobs, Jenkins, Pritzker and Ware, which specialized in the defense of citizens charged with drug-related crimes. He left that firm in 1983 to become a lobbyist for the American Agriculture Movement, an organization that represents farmers and ranchers in rural areas of the United States. In that capacity, he also represented James Nichols, then secretary of agriculture for the state of Minnesota. After working for four years as a lobbyist, Stroup then took a position as executive director of the National Association of Criminal Defense Lawyers (NACDL), a bar association for criminal defense attorneys in the United States, where he remained until 1993. For the next two years, he was employed in Alexandria, Virginia, as staff counsel for the National Center on Institutions and Alternatives (NCIA), an organization that works to keep nonviolent offenders (such as individuals arrested for marijuana possession) out of prison. In 1995, Stroup returned once more to NORML, where he resumed his post as executive director before leaving that post in 2005 to become legal counsel for the organization.

Stroup resigned from his post as executive director at NORML because, as he told the *Post* reporter, he looked in the mirror one morning and saw "this gray-haired old man and I said, 'I think we need younger leadership.'" His replacement at the organization was 39-year-old Allen St. Pierre. Even though he left leadership of the organization he founded, Stroup continues to speak and write about the legalization of marijuana and to defend individuals arrested for marijuana-related crimes.

UN Office On Drugs and Crime

Vienna International Centre
P.O. Box 500
A 1400 Vienna
Austria
Phone: + 43-1-26060
Fax: + 43-1-263-3389
E-mail: info@unodc.org
URL: http://www.unodc.org/

The UN Office on Drugs and Crime (UNODC) was created in 1997 as the Office for Drug Control and Crime Prevention by the merger of two pre-existing United Nations (UN) organizations, the United Nations International Drug Control Programme and the Crime Prevention and Criminal Justice Division of the United Nations office at Vienna, Austria. The organization's name was changed to its present name in 2002. UNODC is one of 32 funds, programs, agencies, departments, and offices that make up the United Nations Development Group (UNDG) and whose goal it is to provide more effective and more efficient support to nations attempting to achieve certain internationally agreed upon development goals. A few other members of the UNDG are the United Nations Children's Fund, United Nations Population Fund, World Food Programme, Office of the High Commissioner for Human Rights, Joint United Nations Programme on HIV/AIDS, and the World Health Organization.

UNODC lists three main "pillars" that underlie its work. The first pillar is research and analysis aimed at improving the world's knowledge about drugs and crime with the goal of providing an accurate basis for the development of policies and legislation. The second pillar is assistance to nations in the development of international treaties and domestic legislation designed to fight drug abuse, crime, and terrorism. The third pillar is field-based cooperative projects that improve the ability of nations to counteract substance abuse, crime, and terrorism.

To accomplish these goals, UNODC is divided administratively into four major divisions for operations, treaty affairs, policy analysis and public affairs, and management. The Division for Operations is responsible for programs such as HIV/AIDS; drug prevention, treatment, and rehabilitation; sustainable livelihoods; and justice. The Division for Treaty Affairs deals with activities such as organized crime and illicit trafficking, corruption and economic crime, and terrorism prevention. The Division for Policy Analysis and Public Affairs is concerned with laboratory and scientific studies, statistics and surveys, studies and threat analysis, strategic planning, and advocacy. The Division of Management is responsible for in-house management issues such as human resources and information technology.

To facilitate its services to member states of the United Nations, UNODC has developed a Menu of Services that clearly and succinctly outlines the ways in which the organization can assist individual nations and regions in dealing with problems of illicit drugs, crime, and terrorism. That Menu of Services is available in print and electronic form, the latter at the agency's website at http://www.unodc.org/documents/frontpage/MoS_book11 _LORES.pdf. Some of the services that are listed and described in the Menu of Services publication are the following:

- Research and threat analysis
- Cross-border cooperation and knowledge sharing
- Statistical expertise
- Quantitative and qualitative trends
- Research and survey reports; threat assessments
- Capacity development assessment
- Expert advice
- Specialized training
- Legal assistance
- Model laws and legislation

- Scientific and forensic services
- Awareness raising campaigns and initiatives

As a way of carrying out its general program, UNODC has developed specific focus areas within which to conduct its day-to-day work. Currently, these focus areas include alternative development; corruption; crime prevention and criminal justice; drug prevention, treatment, and care; drug trafficking; HIV/AIDS; human trafficking and migrant smuggling; money laundering; organized crime; piracy; terrorism prevention; and wildlife and forest crime. An example of the work conducted under these focus topics is the program on drug prevention, treatment, and care. For many years, UNODC has been working to identify best practices in achieving progress in these three areas of substance abuse. As a result of these efforts, it has developed two programs, Global Youth Network against Drug Abuse and the Global Initiative on Primary Prevention of Substance Abuse. The former program is intended to provide a mechanism by which young adults can disseminate throughout the international community knowledge about programs that they have developed. The program's Taking Action website describes some of these programs on topics such as preventing the use of amphetamine-type stimulants among young people, putting the right message across to youth, prevention in school, working with families, alternative activities, working with vulnerable populations, and violence prevention: the evidence. The Global Initiative on Primary Prevention of Substance Abuse was a collaborative project between UNODC and the World Health Organization (WHO), funded by the government of Norway. The program involved identifying successful drug prevention programs in various countries around the world and then providing those programs with training as well as financial and technical support. One result of this effort was the development of a set of practices that have been found to be successful in reducing substance abuse.

UNODC has developed tools for use in its campaign against illicit drugs, crime, and terrorism such as campaigns (World Drug Day, International Day against Drug Abuse and Illicit Trafficking, and International Anti-Corruption Day); commissions (Commission on Narcotic Drugs, Commission on Crime Prevention and Criminal Justice, and Governance and Finance Working Group); an annual Congress on Crime Prevention and Criminal Justice; data and analysis tools (*World Drug Report*, *Global Report on Trafficking in Persons*, statistical reports, transnational organized crime threat assessments, and studies and journals); legal tools (the Legal Library, Human Trafficking Case Law Database, collection of international drugs control conventions and commentaries, Directories of Competent National Authorities, Mutual Legal Assistance Request Writer Tool, and model laws and treaties); and laboratory and forensic science services (information on drug analysis and forensic science laboratories; criminal justice system and law enforcement authorities; regulatory and health authorities, quality assurance support; manuals, guidelines and publications; partnerships; news and events; and synthetic drugs).

UNODC produces many publications that are generally available in both print and electronic format. A few of the most important are the *Bulletin of Narcotics*, which was published between 1949 and 2008, the *Forum on Crime and Society*, which was published between 2001 and 2006, and *World Drug Report*, which has been published annually since 1999 and is one of the best resources on drug statistics currently available.

U.S. Drug Enforcement Administration
Mailstop AES
8701 Morrissette Dr.
Springfield, VA 22152
Phone: (202) 307-1000
E-mail: [none provided]
URL: http://www.justice.gov/dea/index.htm

The U.S. government has had a succession of agencies designed to deal with substance abuse problems in general, and marijuana in particular. The earliest of these agencies was the Narcotics Division, established within the Bureau of Internal Revenue in 1921. The agency was created to carry out mandates of the Harrison Narcotic Act of 1914. A year later, a second agency was created, the Federal Narcotics Control Board, whose mandate it was to make and publish regulations concerning the import and export of narcotic substances. These two agencies were consolidated in 1930 to form the Bureau of Narcotics within the U.S. Department of the Treasury. In yet another reorganization act, the Bureau of Narcotics and the Bureau of Drug Abuse Control (created within the Food and Drug Administration in 1965) were combined to form the Bureau of Narcotics and Dangerous Drugs within the Department of Justice. The final step in this sequence of events occurred on July 28, 1973, when President Richard Nixon signed the Reorganization Plan No. 2 of 1973, bringing under one roof all agencies in the federal government with some responsibility for substance abuse, including the Bureau of Narcotics and Dangerous Drugs and a number of smaller agencies in a variety of cabinet departments. The new agency, which still exists today, was the Drug Enforcement Administration (DEA). The first administrator of the DEA was John R. Bartels, Jr., a former federal prosecutor. The current DEA administrator (as of early 2012) is Michele M. Leonhart, a career DEA agent.

As specified on its website, the mission of the DEA is "to enforce the controlled substances laws and regulations of the United States and bring to the criminal and civil justice system of the United States, or any other competent jurisdiction, those organizations and principal members of organizations, involved in the growing, manufacture, or distribution of controlled substances appearing in or destined for illicit traffic in the United States; and to recommend and support non-enforcement programs aimed at reducing the availability of illicit controlled substances on the domestic and international markets."

DEA activities fall into one of about 20 major categories, including:

• Organized Crime Drug Enforcement Task Forces (OCDETF): This program involves the participation of a number of federal agencies to attack major drug trafficking and money laundering activities related to the importation and sale of illegal drugs to the United States.

• Demand reduction: In addition to apprehending and prosecuting substance abusers and their enablers, the agency works to reduce the use of illegal drugs by working with state, regional, and local agencies to help individuals understand the dangers posed by substance abuse and to find was of avoiding involvement in drug activities.

• Asset forfeiture: Federal law provides that profits from drug-related activities collected by drug enforcement activities are forfeited to the government and may be used to support worthy causes through the Asset Forfeiture Fund.

• Aviation program: Since 1971, the DEA has provided air support for ground activities of the agency's agents, helping to detect, locate, identify, and assess narcotics-related trafficking activities.

• Diversion control: This program is aimed at monitoring and controlling the illegal use of prescription drugs, the fastest growing substance-abuse problem in the United States today. The program involves the arrest of physicians who sell prescriptions to drug dealers, pharmacists who falsify records and sell prescription drugs to dealers, employees who steal from inventories and/or falsify records, and individuals who obtain prescription drugs by illegal activities.

• Forensic sciences: The DEA forensic science laboratory provides assistance to prosecutors who need evidence for the conduct of criminal cases involving the use of illegal substances.

- Foreign cooperative investigations. Since almost all illegal substances (except for marijuana) are grown or produced outside the United States, cooperation with foreign government where drugs are produced is an essential feature of the U.S. drug control program.

The DEA Domestic Cannabis Eradication/Suppression Program (DCE/SP) is of special interest largely because marijuana is the only major schedule I drug grown in the United States. One of the major goals of DCE/SP, then, is to eliminate the supply of marijuana in the United States by finding and destroying farms where the cannabis plant is being grown. In 2010, for example, DEA agents identified and eradicated a total of 23,622 outdoor marijuana growing sites with an estimated total of 9,866,766 individual plants. In addition, 4,721 indoor sites were identified and eradicated, with a loss of 462,419 plants. Total estimated value of all the destroyed plants was $34,311,819. In addition to plant destruction, DEA agents made 9,687 arrests of individuals associated with plant growth and collected 5,081 weapons.

Each year, the DEA schedules special operations to carry out the agency's mission. In 2011, for example, those operations included Operation Fire and Ice, a five-year investigation of an international drug trafficking organization called La Oficina de Envigado based in Medellín, Colombia; Operation Pill Nation, which involved the arrest of 22 individuals and the seizure of more than $2.2 million in cash from rogue pain clinics in South Florida; and the 38th Street Gang Roundup, in which federal agents seized more than seven kilograms of cocaine, one pound of methamphetamine, and about $250,000 cash from a notorious gang located in south Los Angeles.

DEA makes available on its website valuable print and electronic publications, including the biweekly electronic newsletter

Dateline DEA; a set of 33 "Drug Facts" informational sheets; an annual report *Drugs of Abuse*; a publication especially designed for state and local law enforcement officials, environmental protection groups, and public health agencies, *Guidelines for Law Enforcement for the Cleanup of Clandestine Drug Laboratories*; a document dealing with the decriminalization of currently illegal drugs, *Speaking Out against Drug Legalization*; and two technical publications, *Microgram Bulletin* and *Microgram Journal*.

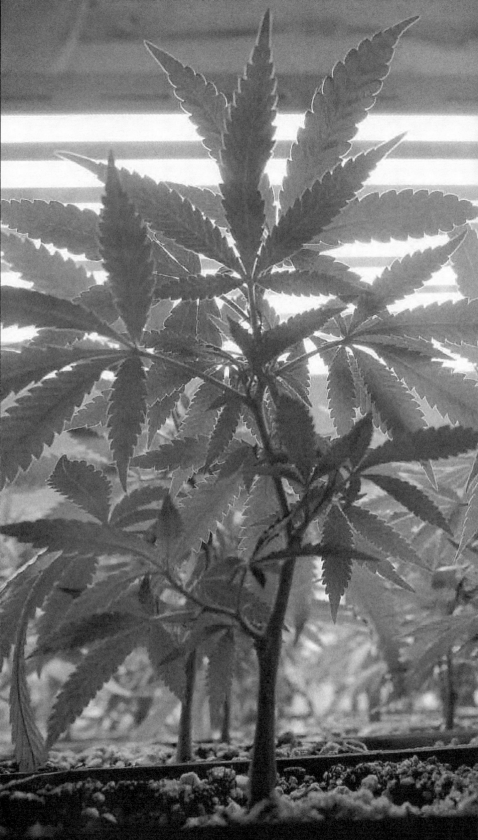

5   Data and Documents

This chapter provides some relevant data and documents dealing with cannabis and related products. The "Data" section provides basic information on current and historical trends in marijuana use as well as arrests in the United States and other parts of the world. The "Documents" section, which follows, is arranged in chronological order and includes excerpts from important committee and commission reports; from bills, acts, and laws; and from important legal cases.

Data

Table 5.1: Marijuana Use in the United States in 2010

Table 5.1 shows the number of Americans in 2010 who used marijuana in one of three ranges—at any time in their lifetime, during the last year, and within the 30 days preceding the survey.

The marijuana plant, *Cannabis sativa*, is the plant most commonly used for recreational and medical purposes. (AP Photo/Ted S. Warren)

Table 5.1 Marijuana Use in the United States in 2010

Characteristic	Lifetime[1]	Past Year[1]	Past Month[1]
TOTAL	106,232	29,206	17,373
Age			
12–17 years old	4,139	3,400	1,796
18–25 years old	17,415	10,161	6,292
26 years and older	84,678	15,645	9,286
Gender			
Male	58,279	17,804	11,212
Female	47,953	11,402	6,161
Hispanic Origin/Race			
Not Hispanic or Latino	94,999	25,295	15,242
White	78,008	19,682	11,880
Black/African American	12,285	4,147	2,599
American Indian/Alaska Native	583	196	121
Native Hawaiian/Pacific Islander	212	50	21
Asian	2,227	627	296
Two or more races	1,683	593	325
Hispanic or Latino	11,233	3,911	2,131

[1]Indicates have used at any time in one's life; within the past year; within the past month.

Source: Results from the 2010 National Survey on Drug Use and Health: Summary of National Findings. Rockville, MD: U.S. Department of Health and Human Services. Substance Abuse and Mental Health Services Administration. Center for Behavioral Health Statistics and Quality, September 2011, Table 1.26A.

Table 5.2: Marijuana-Related Arrests

Table 5.2 provides arrest statistics for two groups of individuals: those arrested for simple possession of marijuana, and those arrested for trafficking in the drug over periods of time ranging from 1980 to 2010 in the former case, and from 1995 to 2010 in the latter case.

Table 5.2   Marijuana-Related Arrests

Year	Trafficking	Possession	All Marijuana	Trafficking	Possession
			Percentage of All Drug Arrests		
1980	63,318	338,664	69.2	10.9	58.3
1990	66,460	260,390	30.0	6.1	23.9
1995	85,614	503,350	39.9	5.8	34.1
1996	94,891	546,751	42.6	6.3	36.3
1997	88,682	606,591	43.9	5.6	38.3
1998	84,191	598,694	43.8	5.4	38.4
1999	85,641	630,626	46.0	5.5	40.5
2000	88,455	646,042	46.5	5.6	40.9
2001	82,519	641,109	45.6	5.2	40.4
2002	83,096	613,896	45.3	5.4	39.9
2003	92,300	662,886	45.0	5.5	39.5
2004	87,329	686,402	42.6	4.9	37.7
2005	90,471	696,074	42.6	4.9	37.7
2006	90,711	738,916	43.9	4.8	39.1
2007	97,583	775,137	47.4	5.3	42.1
2008	93,640	754,224	49.8	5.5	44.3
2009	99,815	758,593	51.6	6.0	45.6
2010	103,247	750,591	52.1	6.3	45.8

Source: "Get the Facts." DrugWars.org. Table information calculated from Federal Bureau of Investigations. *Crime in the United States*, annual publication, 1980–2010. http://www.drugwarfacts.org/cms/Marijuana#Total and http://www.fbi.gov/about-us/cjis/ucr/crime-in-the-u.s/2010/crime-in-the-u.s.-2010. Accessed on September 29, 2012.

Table 5.3: Marijuana Use by Various Categories

Table 5.3 shows marijuana use by U.S. high school students in 2009 by gender, ethnicity, and grade level.

Table 5.3   Marijuana Use by Various Categories

Category	Ever Used Marijuana			Current Marijuana Use[1]		
	Female	Male	Total	Female	Male	Total
Race/Ethnicity						
White	33.7	37.4	35.7	17.9	23.0	20.7
Black	38.0	44.3	41.2	18.7	25.6	22.2
Hispanic	35.6	44.2	39.9	18.2	25.0	21.6
Grade						
9	25.7	26.9	26.4	15.5	15.5	15.5
10	33.0	37.7	35.5	17.9	23.9	21.1
11	39.5	44.3	42.0	19.5	26.7	23.2
12	40.2	50.9	45.6	19.1	29.9	24.6
TOTAL	34.3	39.0	36.8	17.9	23.4	20.8

[1]Use within 30 days prior to survey.

Source: "Youth Risk Behavior Surveillance: United States, 2009." http://www.cdc.gov/mmwr/preview/mmwrhtml/ss5905a1.htm#tab40. Accessed on September 29, 2012.

Table 5.4: Marijuana Use in Europe

Table 5.4 shows the last 30 days' prevalence of drug use by age and country based on the most recent national general population survey available since 2000.

Table 5.4   Marijuana Use in Europe

Country	Year of Survey	Percentage of Users, Ages 15–64 Years		
		Lifetime Use	Last Year Use	Last 30-Day Use
Austria	2008	14.2	3.5	1.7
Belgium	2008	14.3	5.1	3.1
Bulgaria	2008	7.3	2.7	1.4
Croatia	—	—	—	—
Cyprus	2009	11.6	4.4	2.5
Czech Republic	2009	27.6	11.1	4.1

(*continued*)

Table 5.4   (*continued*)

Country	Year of Survey	Percentage of Users, Ages 15–64 Years		
		Lifetime Use	Last Year Use	Last 30-Day Use
Denmark	2010	32.5	5.4	2.3
Estonia	2008	—	6.0	1.4
Finland	2006	14.3	3.6	1.6
France	2005	30.6	8.6	4.8
Germany	2009	25.6	4.8	2.4
Greece	2004	8.9	1.7	0.9
Hungary	2007	8.5	2.3	1.2
Ireland	2007/8	21.9	6.3	2.6
Italy	2008	32.0	14.3	6.9
Latvia	2007	12.1	4.9	1.8
Lithuania	2008	11.9	5.6	1.2
Luxembourg	—	—	—	—
Malta	2001	3.5	0.8	0.5
Netherlands	2005	22.6	5.4	3.3
Norway	2009	14.6	3.8	1.6
Poland	2006	9.0	2.7	0.9
Portugal	2007	11.7	3.6	2.4
Romania	2007	1.5	0.4	0.1
Slovenia	2007	—	3.1	—
Slovakia	2006	16.1	6.9	2.0
Spain	2009	32.1	10.6	7.6
Sweden	2010	14.3	2.8	1.0
Turkey	—	—	—	—
England and Wales	2009–2010	30.6	6.6	3.9

Missing data reflects failure of a nation to report information for the period(s) noted.

Source: European Monitoring Centre for Drugs and Drug Addiction (EMCDDA). *A Cannabis Reader: Global Issues and Local Experiences*, Monograph series 8, Volume 1. Lisbon, Portugal: European Monitoring Centre for Drugs and Drug Addiction, 2008, Tables GPS1, GPS2, and GPS3. Available online at http://www.emcdda.europa.eu/stats11/gpstab1b; http://www.emcdda.europa.eu/stats11/gpstab2a; http://www.emcdda.europa.eu/stats11/gpstab3a.

Table 5.5: Eradication of Cannabis Plants in the United States

Table 5.5 shows the results of the Drug Enforcement Administration's ongoing Cannabis Eradication/Suppression Program for 2010.

Table 5.5   Eradication of Cannabis Plants in the United States[1]

State	Outdoor		Indoor		Total	Arrests	Value
	Sites	Plants	Sites	Plants			
California	1,481	7,204,355	2791	188,297	7,392,652	1,591	$8,261,397
Hawaii	399	96,623	34	719	97,333	119	$303,035
Kentucky	7,434	326,837	94	3,390	330,227	812	$1,079,195
North Carolina	253	131,210	49	1,991	133,201	166	$41,198
Ohio	1,522	84,660	240	20,461	105,121	336	$771,715
Oregon	276	237,909	267	19,941	257,850	430	$1,389,255
Tennessee	2,548	332,987	3	472	333,459	29	$7,200
Utah	47	83,864	2	117	83,981	11	$285,000
Washington	253	573,792	231	35,131	608,923	313	$4,421,775
West Virginia	573	418,891	40	1,219	420,110	173	$50,890

[1] By number of plants destroyed.

Source: Drug Enforcement Administration. 2010 Domestic Cannabis Eradication/suppression Program Statistical Report. http://www.albany.edu/sourcebook/pdf/t4382009.pdf. Accessed on September 29, 2012.

Table 5.6: Attitudes and Practices Concerning Marijuana among U.S. Twelfth Graders

Table 5.6 shows trends in attitudes about and use of marijuana among twelfth grade students in the United States between 1975 and 2011.

Table 5.6   Attitudes and Practices Concerning Marijuana among U.S. Twelfth Graders

	Percentage of "Disapproving"[1]			
Year	Trying Marijuana Once or Twice	Smoking Marijuana Occasionally	Smoking Marijuana Regularly	Used Marijuana within the Past 30 Days
1975	47.0	54.8	71.9	27.1
1976	38.4	47.8	69.5	32.2
1977	33.4	44.3	65.5	35.4
1978	33.4	43.5	67.5	37.1
1979	34.2	45.3	69.2	36.5
1980	39.0	49.7	74.6	33.7
1981	40.0	52.6	77.4	31.6
1982	45.5	59.1	80.6	28.5
1983	46.3	60.7	82.5	27.0
1984	49.3	63.5	84.7	25.2
1985	51.4	65.8	85.5	25.7
1986	54.6	69.0	86.6	23.4
1987	56.6	71.6	89.2	21.0
1988	60.8	74.0	89.3	18.0
1989	64.6	77.2	89.8	16.7
1990	67.8	80.5	91.0	14.0
1991	68.7	79.4	89.3	13.8
1992	69.9	79.7	90.1	11.9
1993	63.3	75.5	87.6	15.5
1994	57.6	68.9	82.3	19.0
1995	56.7	66.7	81.9	21.2
1996	52.5	62.9	80.0	21.9
1997	51.0	63.2	78.8	23.7
1998	51.6	64.4	81.2	22.8

(continued)

Table 5.6   (continued)

| Year | Percentage of "Disapproving"[1] | | | |
	Trying Marijuana Once or Twice	Smoking Marijuana Occasionally	Smoking Marijuana Regularly	Used Marijuana within the Past 30 Days
1999	48.8	62.5	78.6	23.1
2000	52.5	65.8	79.7	21.6
2001	49.1	63.2	79.3	22.4
2002	51.6	63.4	78.3	21.5
2003	53.4	64.2	78.7	21.2
2004	52.7	65.4	80.7	19.9
2005	55.0	67.8	82.0	19.8
2006	55.6	69.3	82.2	18.3
2007	58.6	70.2	83.3	18.8
2008	55.5	67.3	79.6	19.4
2009	54.8	65.6	80.3	20.6
2010	51.6	62.0	77.7	21.4
2011	51.3	60.9	77.5	22.6

[1]Answer alternatives were (1) Don't disapprove, (2) Disapprove, and (3) Strongly disapprove. Percentages are shown for categories (2) and (3) combined.

Source: Johnston, L. D., O'Malley, P. M., Bachman, J. G., & Schulenberg, J. E. (December 14, 2011). "Marijuana use continues to rise among U.S. teens, while alcohol use hits historic lows." University of Michigan News Service: Ann Arbor, MI. Retrieved 01/03/2012 from http://www.monitoringthefuture.org. Used by permission.

Documents

India Hemp Drugs Commission (1895)

In 1893, the British House of Commons, concerned about reported harmful effects of the use of marijuana by Indian natives, commissioned a study of the use of marijuana in India. The report of the commission, issued in 1895, was 3,281 pages long and contained the views of more than 1,200 witnesses from every level of society. The main conclusions reached by the commission were as follows (typographical errors in the cited source have been corrected at †):

552. The Commission have now examined all the evidence before them regarding the effects attributed to hemp drugs. It

will be well to summarize briefly the conclusions to which they come. It has been clearly established that the occasional use of hemp in moderate doses may be beneficial; but this use may be regarded as medicinal in character. It is rather to the popular and common use of the drugs that the Commission will now confine their attention. It is convenient to consider the effects separately as affecting the physical, mental, or moral nature. In regard to the physical effects, the Commission have come to the conclusion that the moderate use of hemp drugs is practically attended by no evil results at all. There may be exceptional cases in which, owing to idiosyncracies of constitution, the drugs in even moderate use may be injurious. There is probably nothing the use of which may not possibly be injurious in cases of exceptional intolerance. There are also many cases where in tracts with a specially malarious climate, or in circumstances of hard work and exposure, the people attribute beneficial effects to the habitual moderate use of these drugs; and there is evidence to show that the popular impression may have some basis in fact. Speaking generally, the Commission are of opinion that the moderate use of hemp drugs appears to cause no appreciable physical injury of any kind. The excessive use does cause injury. As in the case of other intoxicants, excessive use tends to weaken the constitution and to render the consumer more susceptible to disease. In respect to *[†]* particular diseases which according to a *[†]* considerable number of witnesses should be associated directly with hemp drugs, it appears to be reasonably established that the excessive use of these drugs does not cause asthma; that it may indirectly cause dysentery by weakening the constitution as above indicated; and that it may cause bronchitis mainly through the action of the inhaled smoke on the bronchial tubes.

In respect to the alleged mental effects of the drugs, the Commission have come to the conclusion that the moderate use of hemp drugs produces no injurious effects on the mind. It may indeed be accepted that in the case of specially marked neurotic diathesis, even the moderate use may produce mental injury. For the slightest mental stimulation or excitement may have that effect in such cases. But putting aside these quite exceptional cases, the moderate use of these drugs produces no mental injury. It is otherwise with the excessive use. Excessive use indicates and intensifies mental instability. It tends to weaken the mind. It may even lead to insanity. It has been said by Dr. Blanford that "two factors only are necessary for the causation of insanity, which are complementary, heredity, and stress. Both enter into every case: the stronger the influence of one factor, the less of the other factor is requisite to produce the result. Insanity, therefore, needs for its production a certain instability of nerve tissue and the incidence of a certain disturbance." It appears that the excessive use of hemp drugs may, especially in cases where there is any weakness or hereditary predisposition, induce insanity. It has been shown that the effect of hemp drugs in this respect has hitherto been greatly exaggerated, but that they do sometimes produce insanity seems beyond question.

In regard to the moral effects of the drugs, the Commission are of opinion that their moderate use produces no moral injury whatever. There is no adequate ground for believing that it injuriously affects the character of the consumer. Excessive consumption, on the other hand, both indicates and intensifies moral weakness or depravity. Manifest excess leads directly to loss of self-respect, and thus to moral degradation. In respect to his relations with society, however, even the excessive consumer of hemp drugs is ordinarily inoffensive. His excesses may indeed bring him to degraded poverty which may lead him to dishonest practices; and occasionally, but apparently very rarely indeed, excessive indulgence in hemp drugs may lead to violent [†] crime. But for all practical purposes it may be laid down that there is little or no connection between the use of hemp drugs and crime.

Source: Young, W. Mackworth, et al. *Report of the Indian Hemp Drugs Commission, 1893–94.* [n.p.]: Government Central Printing Office, 1894, vol. 1, 263–64. Also available online at http://www.drugtext.org/Table/Indian-Hemp-Commission -Report/.

Marihuana Tax Act (1937)

This act was the first effort by the U.S. government to regulate the use of marijuana, hemp, and other forms of cannabis. It did not actually make such use illegal, but it did assess a tax on the use of such materials. The tax was modest—about $1 for each type of use—but the penalties for not paying the tax were severe. Congress hoped, apparently, to "tax out of existence" the use of cannabis products in the United States.

Section 1 of the act consists of definitions of terms used in the act. The two most important sections of the act are Section 2, which defines the individuals who are required to pay a tax and the amount of the tax, and Section 12, which defines the penalties for non-payment of the tax.

SEC. 2. (a) Every person who imports, manufactures, produces, compounds, sells, deals in, dispenses, prescribes, administers, or gives away marihuana shall (1) within fifteen days after the effective date of this Act, or (2) before engaging after the expiration of such fifteen-day period in any of the above mentioned activities, and (3) thereafter, on or before July 1 of each year, pay the following special taxes respectively:

(1) Importers, manufacturers, and compounders of marihuana, $24 per year.

(2) Producers of marihuana (except those included within subdivision (4) of this subsection), $1 per year, or fraction thereof, during which they engage in such activity.

(3) Physicians, dentists, veterinary surgeons, and other practitioners who distribute, dispense, give away, administer, or prescribe marihuana to patients upon whom they in the course of their professional practice are in attendance, $1 per year or fraction thereof during which they engage in any of such activities.

(4) Any person not registered as an importer, manufacturer, producer, or compounder who obtains and uses marihuana

in a laboratory for the purpose of research, instruction, or analysis, or who produces marihuana for any such purpose, $1 per year, or fraction thereof, during which he engages in such activities.

(5) Any person who is not a physician, dentist, veterinary surgeon, or other practitioner and who deals in, dispenses, or gives away marihuana, $3 per year: Provided, That any person who has registered and paid the special tax as an importer, manufacturer, compounder, or producer, as required by subdivisions (1) and (2) of this subsection, may deal in, dispense, or give away marihuana imported, manufactured, compounded, or produced by him without further payment of the tax imposed by this section.

. . .

SEC. 12. Any person who is convicted of a violation of any provision of this Act shall be fined not more than $2,000 or imprisoned not more than five years, or both, in the discretion of the court.

Source: The Marihuana Tax Act of 1937. Pub. 238, 75th Congress, 50 Stat. 551 (August 2, 1937). Available online at http://www.druglibrary.org/schaffer/hemp/taxact/mjtaxact.htm.

The Marihuana Problem in the City of New York (1944)

In 1939, Mayor Fiorello La Guardia appointed a committee from the New York Academy of Medicine to study "The marihuana problem in the city of New York." The committee's final report dealt with the sociological, medical, psychological, and pharmacological consequences of marijuana use. The committee's major conclusions were as follows:

1. Under the influence of marihuana the basic personality structure of the individual does not change but some of the more superficial aspects of his behavior show alteration.

2. With the use of marihuana the individual experiences increased feelings of relaxation, disinhibition and self-confidence.

3. The new feeling of self-confidence induced by the drug expresses itself primarily through oral rather than through physical activity. There is some indication of a diminution in physical activity.

4. The disinhibition which results from the use of marihuana releases what is latent in the individual's thoughts and emotions but does not evoke responses which would be totally alien to him in his undrugged state.

5. Marihuana not only releases pleasant reactions but also feelings of anxiety.

6. Individuals with a limited capacity for effective experience and who have difficulty in making social contacts are more likely to resort to marihuana than those more capable of outgoing responses.

Source: The LaGuardia Committee Report on Marihuana. Summary and discussion. Available online at http://medical marijuana.procon.org/sourcefiles/laguardia.pdf.

Physical Effects of Marijuana Ingestion (1951)

In 1951, the UN Bulletin of Narcotic Drugs *provided a summary report on marijuana, including an extended section on its physical effects on users. Among the effects reported in the* Bulletin *are the following:*

Motor excitation

Weakening of the power of control

Dissociation of ideas

Hypertrophy of the ego

Delirium

Horror of noise

Notion of time

Notion of space

Deformation of perceptions

Dual personality

Suggestibility

Hallucinations

Acute sensitiveness to sound

Disturbances of the affections

Oneiric ecstasy

Source: Bouquet, J. 1951. "Cannabis (concluded)." *UN Bulletin of Narcotic Drugs* 3(1): 22–45. Available online at http://www.unodc.org/unodc/en/data-and-analysis/bulletin/bulletin_1951-01-01_1_page005.html#s0001.

Leary v. United States, 395 U.S. 6 (1969)

This case is important because it was the first successful test, at the highest level, of the constitutionality of the Marihuana Tax Act of 1937. The syllabus for the case provided here describes the circumstances of the case and the major decisions held unanimously by the Supreme Court. Shortly after the decision was issued, Congress repealed the 1937 act and replaced it with the Controlled Substances Act of 1970.

Petitioner, accompanied by his daughter, son, and two others, on an automobile trip from New York to Mexico, after apparent denial of entry into Mexico, drove back across the International Bridge into Texas, where a customs officer, through a search, discovered some marihuana in the car and on petitioner's daughter's person. Petitioner was indicted under 26 U.S.C. § 4744(a)(2), a subsection of the Marihuana Tax Act, and under 21 U.S.C. § 176a. At petitioner's trial, which resulted in his conviction, petitioner admitted acquiring the marihuana in New York (but said he did not know where it had been grown) and driving with it to Laredo, Texas, thence to the Mexican customs station, and back to the United States. The Marihuana Tax Act levies an occupational tax upon all those who "deal in" the drug, and provides that the taxpayer must register his name and place of business with the Internal Revenue Service. The Act imposes a transfer tax "upon all transfers of marihuana" required to be effected with a written order form, and all except a limited number of clearly lawful transfers must be effected with such a form. The Act further imposes a transfer tax of $1 per ounce on a registered transferee and $100 per ounce on an unregistered transferee. The forms, executed by the transferee, must show the transferor's name and address and the amount of marihuana involved. A copy of the form is "preserved" by the Internal Revenue Service, and the information contained in the form is made available to law enforcement officials. Possession of marihuana is a crime in Texas, where petitioner was arrested, in New York, where petitioner asserted the transfer occurred, and in all the other States. Section 4744(a)(2) prohibits transportation or concealment of marihuana by one who acquired it without having paid the transfer tax, which petitioner conceded that he had not done. Petitioner claimed in his motion for a new trial that his conviction under the Marihuana Tax Act violated his privilege against self-incrimination, and he argues that this Court's subsequent decisions in Marchetti v. United States, 390 U. S. 39, Grosso v. United States, 390 U. S. 62, and Haynes v. United States, 390 U. S. 85, require reversal. The Government contends that the Act's transfer tax provisions do not compel incriminatory disclosures because, as administratively construed and applied, they permit prepayment of the tax only by persons whose activities are otherwise lawful. Title 21 U.S.C. § 176a makes it a crime to transport or facilitate the transportation of illegally imported marihuana, with knowledge of its illegal importation, and provides that a defendant's possession of marihuana shall be deemed sufficient evidence that the marihuana was illegally imported or brought into the United States, and that the defendant knew of the illegal importation or bringing in, unless the defendant explains his possession to the satisfaction of the jury. The trial court instructed the jury that it might find petitioner guilty of violating § 176a (1) solely on petitioner's testimony that the marihuana had been brought back from Mexico into the United States and that, with knowledge of that fact, petitioner had continued to transport it, or (2) partly upon his testimony that he had transported the marihuana from New York to Texas and partly upon the § 176a presumption. Petitioner contends that application of that presumption denied him due process of law.

Held:

1. Petitioner's invocation of the privilege against self-incrimination under the Fifth Amendment provided a full defense to the charge under 26 U.S.C. § 4744(a)(2). Pp. 395 U. S. 12-29.

[The Court then provides five reasons for this decision, the first of which was as follows:]

(a) Since the effect of the Act's terms were such that legal possessors of marihuana were virtually certain to be registrants or exempt from the order form requirement, compliance with the transfer tax provisions would have required petitioner, as one not registered but obliged to obtain an order form, unmistakably to identify himself as a member of a "selective group inherently suspect of criminal activities," and thus those provisions created a "real and appreciable" hazard of incrimination within the meaning of Marchetti, Grosso, and Haynes. Pp. 395 U. S. 16-18.

. . .

2. In the circumstances of this case, the application of that part of the presumption in 21 U.S.C. § 176a which provides that a possessor of marihuana is deemed to know of its unlawful importation denied petitioner due process of law in violation of the Fifth Amendment. Pp. 395 U. S. 29-53.

[The Court provides four explanations for this part of the decision.]

Source: *Leary v. United States*, 395 U. S. 6 (1969). Available online at http://supreme.justia.com/us/395/6/case.html.

Controlled Substances Act (1970)

Leary v. United States *(discussed in the preceding section) essentially invalidated U.S. policy for the control of marijuana production, trade, and use. A replacement for the Marihuana Tax Act of 1937 was passed only a year after the Supreme Court's decision in* Leary v. United States. *The new act was the Controlled Substances Act of 1970, now a part of the U.S. Code, Title 21, Chapter 13. That act established the system of "schedules" for various categories of drugs that is still used by agencies of the U.S. government today. It also provides extensive background information about the domestic and international status of drug abuse efforts. Some of the most relevant sections for the domestic portion of the act are reprinted here.*

Section 801 of the act presents Congress's findings and declarations about controlled substances, with special mention in Section 801a of psychotropic drugs:

§ 801. Congressional findings and declarations: controlled substances

The Congress makes the following findings and declarations:

(1) Many of the drugs included within this subchapter have a useful and legitimate medical purpose and are necessary to maintain the health and general welfare of the American people.

(2) The illegal importation, manufacture, distribution, and possession and improper use of controlled substances have a substantial and detrimental effect on the health and general welfare of the American people.

. . .

(7) The United States is a party to the Single Convention on Narcotic Drugs, 1961, and other international conventions designed to establish effective control over international and domestic traffic in controlled substances.

§ 801a. Congressional findings and declarations: psychotropic substances

The Congress makes the following findings and declarations:

(1) The Congress has long recognized the danger involved in the manufacture, distribution, and use of certain psychotropic substances for nonscientific and nonmedical purposes, and has provided strong and effective legislation to control illicit trafficking and to regulate legitimate uses of psychotropic substances in this country. Abuse of psychotropic substances has become a phenomenon common to many countries, however, and is not confined to national borders. It is, therefore, essential that the United States cooperate with other nations in establishing effective controls over international traffic in such substances.

(2) The United States has joined with other countries in executing an international treaty, entitled the Convention on Psycho—tropic Substances and signed at Vienna, Austria, on February 21, 1971, which is designed to establish suitable controls over the manufacture, distribution, transfer, and use of certain psychotropic substances. The Convention is not self-executing, and the obligations of the United States thereunder may only be performed pursuant to appropriate legislation. It is the intent of the Congress that the amendments made by this Act, together with existing law, will enable the United States to meet all of its obligations under the Convention and that no further legislation will be necessary for that purpose.

. . .

Section 802 deals with definitions used in the act, and section 803 deals with a minor housekeeping issue of financing for the act. Section 811 deals with the attorney general's authority for classifying and declassifying drugs and the manner in which these steps are to be taken. In general:

§ 811. Authority and criteria for classification of substances

(a) Rules and regulations of Attorney General; hearing

The Attorney General shall apply the provisions of this subchapter to the controlled substances listed in the schedules established by section 812 of this title and to any other drug or other substance added to such schedules under this subchapter.

Except as provided in subsections (d) and (e) of this section, the Attorney General may by rule—

(1) add to such a schedule or transfer between such schedules any drug or other substance if he—

(A) finds that such drug or other substance has a potential for abuse, and

(B) makes with respect to such drug or other substance the findings prescribed by subsection (b) of section 812 of this title for the schedule in which such drug is to be placed; or

(2) remove any drug or other substance from the schedules if he finds that the drug or other substance does not meet the requirements for inclusion in any schedule.

. . .

Section (b) provides guidelines for the evaluation of drugs and other substances. The next section, (c), is a key element of the act:
(c) Factors determinative of control or removal from schedules
In making any finding under subsection (a) of this section or under subsection (b) of section 812 of this title, the Attorney General shall consider the following factors with respect to each drug or other substance proposed to be controlled or removed from the schedules:

(1) Its actual or relative potential for abuse.

(2) Scientific evidence of its pharmacological effect, if known.

(3) The state of current scientific knowledge regarding the drug or other substance.

(4) Its history and current pattern of abuse.

(5) The scope, duration, and significance of abuse.

(6) What, if any, risk there is to the public health.

(7) Its psychic or physiological dependence liability.

(8) Whether the substance is an immediate precursor of a substance already controlled under this subchapter.

Section (d) is a lengthy discussion of international aspects of the nation's efforts to control substance abuse. Sections (e) through (h) deal with related, but less important, issues of the control of substance abuse. Section 812 is perhaps of greatest interest to the general reader in that it establishes the system of classifying drugs still used in the United States, along with the criteria for classification and the original list of drugs to be included in each schedule (since greatly expanded):

§ 812. Schedules of controlled substances

(a) Establishment

There are established five schedules of controlled substances, to be known as schedules I, II, III, IV, and V. Such schedules shall initially consist of the substances listed in this section. The schedules established by this section shall be updated and republished on a semiannual basis during the two-year period beginning one year after October 27, 1970, and shall be updated and republished on an annual basis thereafter.

(b) Placement on schedules; findings required

Except where control is required by United States obligations under an international treaty, convention, or protocol, in effect on October 27, 1970, and except in the case of an immediate precursor, a drug or other substance may not be placed in any schedule unless the findings required for such schedule are made with respect to such drug or other substance. The findings required for each of the schedules are as follows:

(1) Schedule I.—

(A) The drug or other substance has a high potential for abuse.

(B) The drug or other substance has no currently accepted medical use in treatment in the United States.

(C) There is a lack of accepted safety for use of the drug or other substance under medical supervision.

(2) Schedule II.—

(A) The drug or other substance has a high potential for abuse.

(B) The drug or other substance has a currently accepted medical use in treatment in the United States or a currently accepted medical use with severe restrictions.

(C) Abuse of the drug or other substances may lead to severe psychological or physical dependence.

(3) Schedule III.—

(A) The drug or other substance has a potential for abuse less than the drugs or other substances in schedules I and II.

(B) The drug or other substance has a currently accepted medical use in treatment in the United States.

(C) Abuse of the drug or other substance may lead to moderate or low physical dependence or high psychological dependence.

(4) Schedule IV.—

(A) The drug or other substance has a low potential for abuse relative to the drugs or other substances in schedule III.

(B) The drug or other substance has a currently accepted medical use in treatment in the United States.

(C) Abuse of the drug or other substance may lead to limited physical dependence or psychological dependence relative to the drugs or other substances in schedule III.

(5) Schedule V.—

(A) The drug or other substance has a low potential for abuse relative to the drugs or other substances in schedule IV.

(B) The drug or other substance has a currently accepted medical use in treatment in the United States.

(C) Abuse of the drug or other substance may lead to limited physical dependence or psychological dependence relative to the drugs or other substances in schedule IV.

(c) Initial schedules of controlled substances

Schedules I, II, III, IV, and V shall, unless and until amended [1] pursuant to section 811 of this title, consist of the following drugs or other substances, by whatever official name, common or usual name, chemical name, or brand name designated: *[The initial list of drugs under each schedule follows.]*

Source: GPO Access. U.S. Code, Title 21, Chapter 13. Sections 801, 801a, 811, and 812.

In the Matter of Marijuana Medical Rescheduling Petition (1988)

In 1972, NORML submitted a petition to the U.S. Drug Enforcement Administration (DEA) asking that marijuana be transferred from schedule I to schedule II under provisions of the Controlled Substances Act of 1970. Sixteen years later, DEA administrative judge Francis L. Young announced his decision on this permission. Young reviewed and commented on the use of marijuana to treat specific medical conditions: cancer, glaucoma, multiple sclerosis, spasticity, and hyperparathyroidism. His general conclusions are as follows:

IX.

CONCLUSION AND RECOMMENDED DECISION

Based upon the foregoing facts and reasoning, the administrative law judge concludes that the provisions of the Act permit and require the transfer of marijuana from Schedule I to Schedule II. The Judge realizes that strong emotions are aroused on both sides of any discussion concerning the use of marijuana. Nonetheless it is essential for this Agency, and its Administrator, calmly and dispassionately to review the evidence of record, correctly apply the law, and act accordingly.

Marijuana can be harmful. Marijuana is abused. But the same is true of dozens of drugs or substances which are listed in Schedule II so that they can be employed in treatment by physicians in proper cases, despite their abuse potential.

Transferring marijuana from Schedule I to Schedule II will not, of course, make it immediately available in pharmacies throughout the country for legitimate use in treatment. Other government authorities, Federal and State, will doubtless have to act before that might occur. But this Agency is not charged with responsibility, or given authority, over the myriad other regulatory decisions that may be required before marijuana can actually be legally available. This Agency is charged merely with determining the placement of marijuana pursuant to the provisions of the Act. Under our system of laws the responsibilities of other regulatory bodies are the concerns of those bodies, not of this Agency, [sic]

There are those who, in all sincerity, argue that the transfer of marijuana to Schedule II will "send a signal" that marijuana is "OK" generally for recreational use. This argument is specious. It presents no valid reason for refraining from taking an action required by law in light of the evidence. If marijuana should be placed in Schedule II, in obedience to the law, then that is where marijuana should be placed, regardless of misinterpretation of the placement by some. The reasons for the placement can, and should, be clearly explained at the time the action is taken. The fear of sending such a signal cannot be permitted to override the legitimate need, amply demonstrated in this record, of countless suffers for the relief marijuana can provide when prescribed by a physician in a legitimate case.

The evidence in this record clearly shows that marijuana has been accepted as capable of relieving the distress of great numbers of very ill people, and doing so with safety under medical supervision. It would be unreasonable, arbitrary and capricious for DEA to continue to stand between those sufferers and the benefits of this substance in light of the evidence in this record.

The administrative law judge recommends that the Administrator conclude that the marijuana plant considered as a whole has a currently accepted medical use in treatment in the United States, that there is no lack of accepted safety for use of it under medical supervision and that it may lawfully be transferred from Schedule I to Schedule II. The judge recommends that the Administrator transfer marijuana from Schedule I to Schedule II.

Source: In the Matter of Marijuana Rescheduling Petition. Docket No. 86-22. Available online at http://www.druglibrary .org/olsen/MEDICAL/YOUNG/young1.html.

Gonzales, Attorney General et al. v. Raich et al., 545 U.S. 1 (2005)

Voters in California approved Proposition 215, permitting the use of marijuana for medical purposes, in 1996. An obvious problem created by that action was possible conflict between the new permissive state law and federal law, which prohibits the use of marijuana for any purpose whatsoever. When two California women, Angel Raich and Diane Monson, had their marijuana stashes confiscated by federal officials in 2002, the two filed suit against the attorney general of the United States, John Ashcroft. (Ashcroft was replaced by Alberto Gonzalez as attorney general in 2005, thus accounting for the final title of the case.) The petitioners' case was that the seized marijuana had been grown in the state of California and was used only within the state; the federal government had, therefore, no basis for taking action in the matter. The federal government claimed that there was a possibility that the marijuana being grown in California might be sold or transported out of the state, and therefore the federal government had authority over the case because of the Commerce Clause of the U.S. Constitution. The court ruled in favor of the government by a 6 to 3 vote. In their decision, the majority relied heavily on a 1942 case, Wickard v. Filburn (317 U.S. 111), which established the right of the federal government to control wheat grown by a farmer in Ohio strictly for his own use. The main elements of the decision and the dissenting opinions are as follows (Citations are omitted and indicated by ellipses in braces: { . . . }):
For the majority:

Respondents in this case do not dispute that passage of the CSA [Controlled Substances Act of 1970], as part of the

Comprehensive Drug Abuse Prevention and Control Act, was well within Congress' commerce power. . . . Nor do they contend that any provision or section of the CSA amounts to an unconstitutional exercise of congressional authority. Rather, respondents' challenge is actually quite limited; they argue that the CSA's categorical prohibition of the manufacture and possession of marijuana as applied to the intrastate manufacture and possession of marijuana for medical purposes pursuant to California law exceeds Congress' authority under the Commerce Clause.

[The court next shows how the issue in the present case is similar to the one posed in Wickard v. Filburn.*]*

Even respondents acknowledge the existence of an illicit market in marijuana; indeed, Raich has personally participated in that market, and Monson expresses a willingness to do so in the future. More concretely, one concern prompting inclusion of wheat grown for home consumption in the 1938 Act was that rising market prices could draw such wheat into the interstate market, resulting in lower market prices. *[The court cites* Wickard v. Filburn *here.]* The parallel concern making it appropriate to include marijuana grown for home consumption in the CSA is the likelihood that the high demand in the interstate market will draw such marijuana into that market. While the diversion of homegrown wheat tended to frustrate the federal interest in stabilizing prices by regulating the volume of commercial transactions in the interstate market, the diversion of homegrown marijuana tends to frustrate the federal interest in eliminating commercial transactions in the interstate market in their entirety. In both cases, the regulation is squarely within Congress' commerce power because production of the commodity meant for home consumption, be it wheat or marijuana, has a substantial effect on supply and demand in the national market for that commodity

[An important element in the dissents written by Justices O'Connor, Thomas, and Rehnquist leaned heavily on states' rights arguments. For example, Justice O'Connor writes:]

We enforce the "outer limits" of Congress' Commerce Clause authority not for their own sake, but to protect historic spheres of state sovereignty from excessive federal encroachment and thereby to maintain the distribution of power fundamental to our federalist system of government. . . . One of federalism's chief virtues, of course, is that it promotes innovation by allowing for the possibility that "a single courageous State may, if its citizens choose, serve as a laboratory; and try novel social and economic experiments without risk to the rest of the country." . . . This case exemplifies the role of States as laboratories. The States' core police powers have always included authority to define criminal law and to protect the health, safety, and welfare of their citizens. . . . Exercising those powers, California (by ballot initiative and then by legislative codification) has come to its own conclusion about the difficult and sensitive question of whether marijuana should be available to relieve severe pain and suffering. Today the Court sanctions an application of the federal Controlled Substances Act that extinguishes that experiment, without any proof that the personal cultivation, possession, and use of marijuana for medicinal purposes, if economic activity in the first place, has a substantial effect on interstate commerce and is therefore an appropriate subject of federal regulation.

[Justice Thomas offered an even more strongly worded dissent on the same basis.]

Respondents' local cultivation and consumption of marijuana is not "Commerce . . . among the several States." . . . By holding that Congress may regulate activity that is neither interstate nor commerce under the Interstate Commerce Clause, the Court abandons any attempt to enforce the Constitution's limits on federal power.

. . .

If the Federal Government can regulate growing a half-dozen cannabis plants for personal consumption (not because it is interstate commerce, but because it is inextricably bound up with interstate commerce), then Congress' Article I powers—as expanded by the Necessary and Proper Clause—have no meaningful limits.

...

If the majority is to be taken seriously, the Federal Government may now regulate quilting bees, clothes drives, and potluck suppers throughout the 50 States. This makes a mockery of Madison's assurance to the people of New York that the "powers delegated" to the Federal Government are "few and defined," while those of the States are "numerous and indefinite."

Source: *Gonzales v. Raich*, 545 U.S. 1 (2005). Available online at http://supreme.justia.com/us/545/03-1454/case.html.

Interpretation of Listing of "Tetrahydrocannabinols" in Schedule I 21 CFR Part 1308 [DEA–204] RIN 1117–AA55 (2001)

In 2001, the U.S. Drug Enforcement Administration (DEA) issued a group of three rules reinterpreting the regulation of any product containing THC. In essence, the new rules prohibited the growing, importation, or use of any cannabis product that contains any level of THC whatsoever. This regulation is considerably more severe than earlier interpretations of the Controlled Substances Act of 1970. The regulations were later overturned by a decision of the Ninth Circuit Court of Appeals (whose decision follows) in 2003.

SUMMARY: For the reasons provided herein, the Drug Enforcement Administration (DEA) interprets the Controlled Substances Act (CSA) and DEA regulations to declare any product that contains any amount of tetrahydrocannabinols (THC) to be a schedule I controlled substance, even if such product is made from portions of the cannabis plant that are excluded from the CSA definition of "marihuana."

[The DEA next provides a lengthy justification for the action is taking in this rule, followed by this conclusion:]

Conclusion

By stating that "any material, compound, mixture, or preparation, which contains any quantity of * * * Tetrahydrocannabinols" is a schedule I controlled substance, the plain language of the CSA leads to the conclusion that all products containing any amount of THC are schedule I controlled substances. The legislative history supports this conclusion by revealing that Congress wrote the definition of marijuana intending to control all parts of the cannabis plant that were believed to contain THC. When the CSA was enacted, the implementing regulations did not simply adopt, verbatim, the prior regulations that were expressly limited to synthetic forms of THC. Rather, the word "Tetrahydrocannabinols" was inserted in the regulations at the top of the listing, thereby including all forms of THC (natural and synthetic). DEA therefore interprets the CSA and DEA regulations such that any product that contains any amount of THC is a schedule I controlled substance, even if such product is made from portions of the cannabis plant that are excluded from the definition of marijuana. DEA recognizes that this interpretive rule, standing alone, would effectively prohibit the use of an assortment of industrial products made from the cannabis plant (such as certain paper products, fiber, rope, and animal feed) that Congress intended to allow under the 1937 Marihuana Tax Act. Although the intent of the now-repealed 1937 Act is no longer controlling, DEA is issuing today, in a separate Federal Register document that accompanies this document, an interim rule that will except from CSA control the types of industrial products that were allowed under the 1937 Act, provided such products do not cause THC to enter the human body. See [insert Federal Register cite for interim rule *{The rule mentioned here is found at 21 CFR Part 1308, page 51539; http://frwebgate.access.gpo.gov/cgi-bin/getdoc.cgi?dbname=2001_register&docid=01-25024-filed.pdf}*]. As explained further in the interim rule, all other products made from any of the excluded portions of the cannabis plant (such as edible "hemp" products) remain controlled substances if they cause THC to enter the human body.

Source: "Interpretation of Listing of 'Tetrahydrocannabinols' in Schedule I." *Federal Register* 66(195), October 9,

2001. Rules and Regulations, 51530, 51533. Available online at http://www.justice.gov/dea/pubs/pressrel/final_rules_dea -205f_and_206f.pdf.

Hemp Industries Association et al. v. Drug Enforcement Administration, 333 F.3d 1082 (2003)

The DEA's listing of new rules for the regulation of cannabis, outlined in the preceding document, was challenged by a group of companies including Hemp Industries Association; All-One-God-Faith, Inc. (dba Dr. Bronner's Magic Soaps); Atlas Corporation; Nature's Path.

Foods USA, Inc.; Hemp Oil Canada, Inc.; Hempzels, Inc.; Kenex Ltd.; and Tierra Madre, LLC. The case was argued and decided in two parts, called Hemp I and Hemp II. The court's final decision about the DEA's action as outlined in Hemp II included the following conclusion. (Citations are omitted and indicated by ellipses in braces: { . . . }.)

[7] Congress was aware of the presence of trace amounts of psychoactive agents (later identified as THC) in the resin of non-psychoactive hemp when it passed the 1937 "Marihuana Tax Act," and when it adopted the Tax Act marijuana definition in the CSA. As a result, when Congress excluded from the definition of marijuana "mature stalks of such plant, fiber . . . [and] oil or cake made from the seeds," it also made an exception to the exception, and included "resin extracted from" the excepted parts of the plant in the definition of marijuana, despite the stalks and seeds exception { . . . }. Congress knew what it was doing, and its intent to exclude non-psychoactive hemp from regulation is entirely clear. The DEA's Final Rules are inconsistent with the unambiguous meaning of the CSA definitions of marijuana and THC, and the DEA did not use the appropriate scheduling procedures to add non-psychoactive hemp to the list of controlled substances.

[The court then notes that it has already determined in Hemp I that nonpsychoactive hemp is not banned under schedule I.]

We find unambiguous Congress' intent with regard to the regulation of non-psychoactive hemp. Therefore, we reject the Final Rules at step one of the Chevron test and need not reach Chevron step two. *["Chevron" refers to a case whose precedent is cited in this decision.]*

IV. CONCLUSION

[9] The DEA's Final Rules purport to regulate foodstuffs containing "natural and synthetic THC." And so they can: in keeping with the definitions of drugs controlled under Schedule I of the CSA, the Final Rules can regulate foodstuffs containing natural THC if it is contained within marijuana, and can regulate synthetic THC of any kind. But they cannot regulate *naturally-occurring* THC *not* contained within or derived from marijuana—i.e., non-psychoactive hemp products—because non-psychoactive hemp is not included in Schedule I. The DEA has no authority to regulate drugs that are not scheduled, and it has not followed procedures required to schedule a substance.

[10] The DEA's definition of "THC" contravenes the unambiguously expressed intent of Congress in the CSA and cannot be upheld. DEA-205F and DEA-206F *[The two new rules proposed by the DEA]* are thus scheduling actions that would place non-psychoactive hemp in Schedule I for the first time. In promulgating the Final Rules, the DEA did not follow the procedures in §§ 811(a) and 812(b) of the CSA required for scheduling. The amendments to 21 C.F.R. § 1308.11(d)(27) that make THC applicable to all parts of the Cannabis plant are therefore void. We grant Appellants' petition and permanently enjoin enforcement of the Final Rules with respect to non-psychoactive hemp or products containing it.

Source: *Hemp Industries Association v. DEA*. 333 F.3d 1082. Available online at http://archive.ca9.uscourts.gov/ca9/new opinions.nsf/90DC066FE8E8955688256E31007ACE3B/ $file/0371366.pdf?openelement.

FDA Statement on Health Effects of Marijuana (2006)

By the early 2000s, many claims were being made about the medical benefits of smoking marijuana. At that point, the U.S. Food and Drug Administration (FDA) apparently felt it necessary to issue a statement about these claims. On April 20, 2006, the agency issued the following news release on the medical benefits of marijuana.

Claims have been advanced asserting smoked marijuana has a value in treating various medical conditions. Some have argued that herbal marijuana is a safe and effective medication and that it should be made available to people who suffer from a number of ailments upon a doctor's recommendation, even though it is not an approved drug.

Marijuana is listed in schedule I of the Controlled Substances Act (CSA), the most restrictive schedule. The Drug Enforcement Administration (DEA), which administers the CSA, continues to support that placement and FDA concurred because marijuana met the three criteria for placement in Schedule I under 21 U.S.C. 812(b)(1) (e.g., marijuana has a high potential for abuse, has no currently accepted medical use in treatment in the United States, and has a lack of accepted safety for use under medical supervision). Furthermore, there is currently sound evidence that smoked marijuana is harmful. A past evaluation by several Department of Health and Human Services (HHS) agencies, including the Food and Drug Administration (FDA), Substance Abuse and Mental Health Services Administration (SAMHSA) and National Institute for Drug Abuse (NIDA), concluded that no sound scientific studies supported medical use of marijuana for treatment in the United States, and no animal or human data supported the safety or efficacy of marijuana for general medical use. There are alternative FDA-approved medications in existence for treatment of many of the proposed uses of smoked marijuana.

FDA is the sole Federal agency that approves drug products as safe and effective for intended indications. The Federal Food, Drug, and Cosmetic (FD&C) Act requires that new drugs be shown to be safe and effective for their intended use before being marketed in this country. FDA's drug approval process requires well-controlled clinical trials that provide the necessary scientific data upon which FDA makes its approval and labeling decisions. If a drug product is to be marketed, disciplined, systematic, scientifically conducted trials are the best means to obtain data to ensure that drug is safe and effective when used as indicated. Efforts that seek to bypass the FDA drug approval process would not serve the interests of public health because they might expose patients to unsafe and ineffective drug products. FDA has not approved smoked marijuana for any condition or disease indication.

A growing number of states have passed voter referenda (or legislative actions) making smoked marijuana available for a variety of medical conditions upon a doctor's recommendation. These measures are inconsistent with efforts to ensure that medications undergo the rigorous scientific scrutiny of the FDA approval process and are proven safe and effective under the standards of the FD&C Act. Accordingly, FDA, as the federal agency responsible for reviewing the safety and efficacy of drugs, DEA as the federal agency charged with enforcing the CSA, and the Office of National Drug Control Policy, as the federal coordinator of drug control policy, do not support the use of smoked marijuana for medical purposes.

Source: Inter-Agency Advisory Regarding Claims That Smoked Marijuana Is a Medicine. Available online at http://www.fda.gov/NewsEvents/Newsroom/PressAnnouncements/2006/ucm108643.htm.

Marijuana Abuse (2010)

In 2002, the U.S. National Institute on Drug Abuse issued a report that claimed to present our current knowledge of marijuana abuse and its harmful effects. That report was revised and reissued in September 2010. Some of the major conclusions presented in the report are as follows (internal citations in the document have been omitted):

Effects on the Brain

As THC enters the brain, it causes the user to feel euphoric—or high— . . .

Along with euphoria, relaxation is another frequently reported effect in human studies. Other effects, which vary dramatically among different users, include heightened sensory perception (e.g., brighter colors), laughter, altered perception of time, and increased appetite. After a while, the euphoria subsides, and the user may feel sleepy or depressed. Occasionally, marijuana use may produce anxiety, fear, distrust, or panic.

Marijuana use impairs a person's ability to form new memories (omitted citation) and to shift focus. THC also disrupts coordination and balance by binding to receptors in the cerebellum and basal ganglia—parts of the brain that regulate balance, posture, coordination, and reaction time. Therefore, learning, doing complicated tasks, participating in athletics, and driving are also affected.

Marijuana users who have taken large doses of the drug may experience an acute psychosis, which includes hallucinations, delusions, and a loss of the sense of personal identity. . . .

An enduring question in the field is whether individuals who quit marijuana, even after long-term, heavy use, can recover some of their cognitive abilities. . . .

Effects on General Physical Health

Within a few minutes after inhaling marijuana smoke, an individual's heart rate speeds up, the bronchial passages relax and become enlarged, and blood vessels in the eyes expand, making the eyes look red. The heart rate—normally 70 to 80 beats per minute—may increase by 20 to 50 beats per minute, or may even double in some cases. Taking other drugs with marijuana can amplify this effect.

Limited evidence suggests that a person's risk of heart attack during the first hour after smoking marijuana is four times his or her usual risk. . . .

The smoke of marijuana, like that of tobacco, consists of a toxic mixture of gases and particulates, many of which are known to be harmful to the lungs. Someone who smokes marijuana regularly may have many of the same respiratory problems that tobacco smokers do, such as daily cough and phlegm production, more frequent acute chest illnesses, and a greater risk of lung infections. . . .

In addition, marijuana has the *potential* to promote cancer of the lungs and other parts of the respiratory tract because it contains irritants and carcinogens—up to 70 percent more than tobacco smoke. . . .

A significant body of research demonstrates negative effects of THC on the function of various immune cells, both in vitro in cells and in vivo with test animals. . . .

Is There a Link Between Marijuana Use and Mental Illness?

. . . The strongest evidence to date suggests a link between cannabis use and psychosis (omitted citation). . . . Marijuana use also worsens the course of illness in patients with schizophrenia and can produce a brief psychotic reaction in some users that fades as the drug wears off. . . .

In addition to the observed links between marijuana use and schizophrenia, other less consistent associations have been reported between marijuana use and depression, anxiety, suicidal thoughts among adolescents, and personality disturbances. . . .

Is Marijuana Addictive?

Long-term marijuana use can lead to addiction; that is, people have difficulty controlling their drug use and cannot stop even though it interferes with many aspects of their lives. It is estimated that 9 percent of people who use marijuana will become dependent on it. The number goes up to about 1 in 6 in those who start using young (in their teens) and to 25–50 percent among daily users. . . .

How Does Marijuana Use Affect School, Work, and Social Life?

Research has shown that marijuana's negative effects on attention, memory, and learning can last for days or weeks after the acute effects of the drug wear off (omitted citation). Consequently, someone who smokes marijuana daily may be functioning at a reduced intellectual level most or all of the time. . . .

Does Marijuana Use Affect Driving?

Because marijuana impairs judgment and motor coordination and slows reaction time, an intoxicated person has an increased chance of being involved in and being responsible for an accident. . . .

Can Marijuana Use during Pregnancy Harm the Baby?

Animal research suggests that the body's endocannabinoid system plays a role in the control of brain maturation, particularly in the development of emotional responses. It is conceivable that even low concentrations of THC, when administered during the perinatal period, could have profound and long-lasting consequences for both brain and behavior . . .

Source: *Marijuana Abuse*. Washington, DC: National Institute on Drug Abuse, October 2002; revised September 2010.

States' Medical Marijuana Patient Protection Act (H.R. 1983) (2011)

In 2011, Representative Barney Frank (D-MA) introduced two bills into the U.S. House of Representatives, one removing criminal penalties for the use of marijuana, and one with the same purpose and declaring that federal law shall not prevent individual states from allowing the medical use of marijuana. An excerpt from the latter bill follows:

SEC. 2. CONTROLLED SUBSTANCES ACT.

(a) SCHEDULE.—

(1) Not later than 6 months after the date of enactment of this Act, the Secretary of Health and Human Services, in cooperation with the National Academy of Sciences' Institute of Medicine, shall submit to the Administrator of the Drug Enforcement Administration a recommendation on the listing of marijuana within the Controlled Substances Act (CSA), and shall recommend a listing other than "Schedule I" or "Schedule II."

(2) Not later than 12 months after the date of enactment of this Act, the Administrator of the Drug Enforcement Administration shall, based upon the recommendation of the National Academy of Sciences, issue a notice of proposed rulemaking for the rescheduling of marijuana within the CSA, which shall include a recommendation to list marijuana as other than a "Schedule I" or "Schedule II" substance.

(b) LIMITATIONS ON THE APPLICATION OF THE CONTROLLED SUBSTANCES ACT.—

(1) IN GENERAL.—No provision of the Controlled Substances Act shall prohibit or otherwise restrict in a State in which the medical use of marijuana is legal under State law—

(A) the prescription or recommendation of marijuana for medical use by a medical professional or the certification by a medical professional that a patient has a condition for which marijuana may have therapeutic benefit;

(B) an individual from obtaining, manufacturing, possessing, or transporting within their State marijuana for medical purposes, provided the activities are authorized under State law; or

(C) a pharmacy or other entity authorized under local or State law to distribute medical marijuana to individuals authorized to possess medical marijuana under State law from obtaining, possessing or distributing marijuana to such individuals.

(2) PRODUCTION.—No provision of the Controlled Substances Act shall prohibit or otherwise restrict an entity authorized by a State or local government, in a State in which the possession and use of marijuana for medical purposes is legal from producing, processing, or distributing marijuana for such purposes.

SEC. 3. FEDERAL FOOD, DRUG, AND COSMETIC ACT.

(a) IN GENERAL.—No provision of the Federal Food, Drug, and Cosmetic Act shall prohibit or otherwise restrict in a State in which the medical use of marijuana is legal under State law—

(1) the prescription or recommendation of marijuana for medical use by a medical professional or the certification by a medical professional that a patient has a condition for which marijuana may have therapeutic benefit;

(2) an individual from obtaining, manufacturing, possessing, or transporting within their State marijuana for medical purposes, provided the activities are authorized under State law; or

(3) a pharmacy or other entity authorized under local or State law to distribute medical marijuana to individuals authorized to possess medical marijuana under State law from obtaining, possessing, or distributing marijuana to such individuals.

(b) PRODUCTION.—No provision of the Federal Food, Drug, and Cosmetic Act shall prohibit or otherwise restrict an entity authorized by a State or local government, in a State in which the possession and use of marijuana for medical purposes is legal from producing, processing, or distributing marijuana for such purpose.

SEC. 4. RELATION OF ACT TO CERTAIN PROHIBITIONS RELATING TO SMOKING.

This Act does not affect any Federal, State, or local law regulating or prohibiting smoking in public.

Source: 112th Congress. 1st Session. H. R. 1983. Available online at http://www.gpo.gov/fdsys/pkg/BILLS-112hr1983 ih/pdf/BILLS-112hr1983ih.pdf.

Ending Federal Marijuana Prohibition Act (H.R. 2306) (2011)

The second bill introduced by Representative Frank and Representative Ron Paul (R-TX) was very short, running about one page. Its major section read as follows:

SEC. 2. APPLICATION OF THE CONTROLLED SUBSTANCES ACT TO MARIHUANA.

Part A of the Controlled Substances Act (21 U.S.C. 801 et seq.) is amended by adding at the end the following:

"SEC. 103. APPLICATION OF THIS ACT TO MARIHUANA.

"(a) Prohibition on Certain Shipping or Transportation- This Act shall not apply to marihuana, except that it shall be unlawful only to ship or transport, in any manner or by any means whatsoever, marihuana, from one State, Territory, or District of the United States, or place noncontiguous to but subject to the jurisdiction thereof, into any other State, Territory, or District of the United States, or place noncontiguous to but subject to the jurisdiction thereof, or from any foreign country into any State, Territory, or District of the United States, or place noncontiguous to but subject to the jurisdiction thereof, when such marihuana is intended, by any person interested therein, to be received, possessed, sold, or in any manner used, either in the original package or otherwise, in violation of any law of such State, Territory, or District of the United States, or place non-contiguous to but subject to the jurisdiction thereof.

Source: 112th Congress. 1st Session. H. R. 2306. Available online at http://www.govtrack.us/congress/billtext.xpd?bill =h112-2306.

Marijuana Availability in the United States (2011)

Each year, the National Drug Intelligence Center (NDIC) of the U.S. Department of Justice publishes a report, National Drug Threat Assessment, *which reviews the current status of various illegal drugs in the United States and the prospect for those drugs in coming years. The 2011 report for marijuana is summarized here. Footnotes and references are omitted.*

The availability of marijuana is high in the United States. This is due to steady marijuana production in Mexico—the primary foreign source of marijuana. Further, NDIC believes that high and increasing levels of domestic eradication could be one indicator of increasing domestic production, fueling availability. In contrast, imports of high-grade marijuana from Canada appear to be decreasing as producers shift operations to the U.S. side of the border.

- An estimated 12,000 hectares of cannabis were cultivated in Mexico, and approximately 21,500 metric tons of marijuana were potentially produced during 2008, compared with just 5,600 hectares and 10,100 metric tons in 2005. This estimate represents a 113 percent increase in potential marijuana production since 2005 and a 36 percent increase since 2007.

- During 2008 and 2009, the Government of Mexico (GOM) de-emphasized eradication in favor of focusing counternarcotic resources on interdiction and the targeting of TCO leadership. This change in focus has resulted in less cannabis eradication and potentially more marijuana production.

• Significantly more marijuana was seized entering the United States from Mexico during 2009 and 2010 than in prior years.

Domestic marijuana production is expansive and increasing, especially cultivation by organized groups. The increase in domestic cultivation is fueled by high profitability and demand.

• According to the Domestic Cannabis Eradication/Suppression Program (DCE/SP), a near record 10.3 million plants were eradicated nationally in 2010—approximately 2 million more than in 2008.

• Marijuana production requires little investment and produces large profits; marijuana costs approximately $75 per pound to produce and can be sold for up to $6,000 per pound at the wholesale level, depending on the quality of the processed marijuana.

Outdoor cannabis cultivation on public lands is increasing.

• Data from the U.S. Forest Service (USFS) and Department of Interior (DOI) indicate that a combined total of 4,571,577 plants (44 percent of all cannabis eradicated nationally) were eradicated from federal lands during 2010.

• According to the USFS, the number of plants eradicated from national forests increased dramatically in each of the past 5 years, reaching a new record for eradication in 2010 (3,549,641 plants). Moreover, the number of national forests where grow sites were eradicated increased from approximately 55 forests in 2008 to 59 forests in 2009.

• National forests in California account for the largest plant eradication total from public lands in any region. These national forests also account for the largest increase in the number of eradicated plants on public lands. This increase is in part due to intensified outdoor eradication operations, such as Operation Save Our Sierras in California in 2009 and Operation Trident in 2010.

In 2010, almost all (3,101,765 of 3,549,641 plants) of the cannabis eradicated from national forests was eradicated from 16 national forests in California.

Source: U.S. Department of Justice. National Drug Intelligence Center. *National Drug Threat Assessment.* [n.p.] August 2011, 29–30.

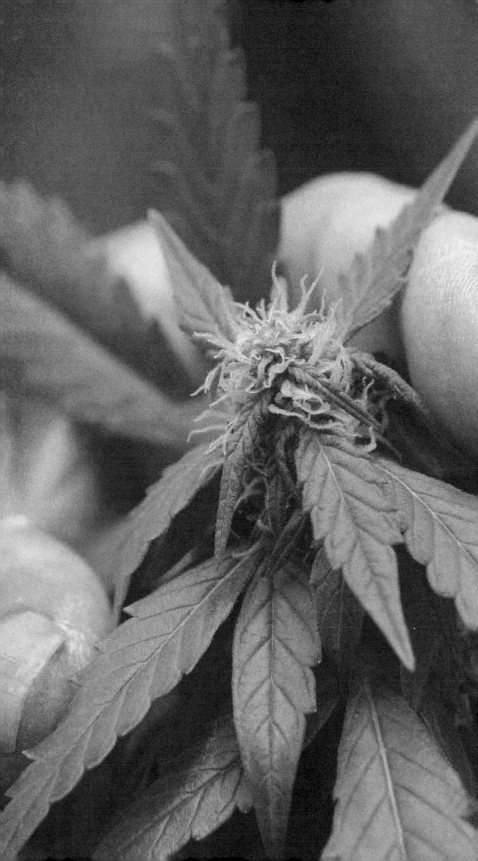

6 Resources

Marijuana is a contentious issue about which volumes have been written in books, articles, reports, pamphlets, brochures, white papers, and other print documents, as well as on the Internet. Many of these resources provide relatively unbiased information on the history of cannabis, its physical and psychological effects, and efforts to establish legal controls (or to remove such controls) over the centuries. This chapter provides a sampling of that literature. The chapter is divided into two major sections, print resources and nonprint resources. In turn, print resources are further divided into three subsections: books, articles, and reports. Given the ubiquity of Internet references today, some items could be assigned to more than one category and where that is possible, it is so noted in the listing. The reader should be aware that a large body of research is now available on the physical, mental, emotional, and moral effects of cannabis use that often produces ambiguous and contradictory results. The studies list here must be regarded as no more than the tip of the iceberg of this research.

The highest concentration of THC in a marijuana plant is found in its buds. (AP Photo/Rich Pedroncelli)

Print Resources

Books

Anderson, Patrick. *High in America: The True Story Behind NORML and the Politics of Marijuana.* New York: Viking Press, 1981.

Anderson presents a detailed and fascinating story about one of the major groups fighting for the decriminalization of marijuana use in the United States. The book is also available in full online at http://www.druglibrary.org/special/anderson/highinamerica1.htm.

Barbour, Scott. *Should Marijuana Be Legalized?* San Diego, CA: ReferencePoint Press, 2011.

This book for young adults presents all sides of the question of the legalization of marijuana.

Bello, Joan. *The Benefits of Marijuana: Physical, Psychological, and Spiritual,* final edition *[sic]*. Susquehanna, PA: Lifeservices Press, 2008.

After an introductory section on the effects of marijuana on the body, the author turns her attention to the physical, psychological, and spiritual benefits of using the drug, along with discussions of specific conditions for which it can be used and legal problems associated with its use.

Bjornlund, Lydia D. *Marijuana.* San Diego, CA: ReferencePoint Press, 2012.

This book is intended for juvenile readers. It reviews both social and economic arguments for and against legalizing marijuana and raises the question as to whether the drug's medical benefits justify legalization.

Boire, Richard Glen, and Kevin Feeney. *Medical Marijuana Law.* Oakland, CA: Ronin Publishing, 2006.

This book provides a complete (if somewhat outdated) discussion of all legal aspects relating to the use of marijuana for medical purposes such as definition of terms involved, basic legal issues, qualifying conditions for use of the drug, finding a doctor with whom to work, forms of medical marijuana, patient rights and responsibilities, physician rights and responsibilities, and medical marijuana statutes.

Bonnie, Richard J., and Charles H. Whitebread. *The Marijuana Conviction: A History of Marijuana Prohibition in the United States.* New York: Lindesmith Center, 1999.

This edition is a reprint of the original 1974 book, now widely considered to be one of the great classics in the literature of marijuana criminalization. The book describes in well-written detail the process by which marijuana went from a highly regarded medical substance to a banned drug in the United States.

Booth, Martin. *Cannabis: A History.* New York: Picador Press, 2005.

The author follows the long history of marijuana use, with special attention to the process by which it was transformed from a respected and widely used substance into an illegal drug.

Carter, Gregory T., Dale Gieringer, and Ed Rosenthal. *Marijuana Medical Handbook: Practical Guide to Therapeutic Uses of Marijuana*, revised edition. Oakland, CA: Quick American Archives, 2008.

This book deals with issues related to the use of medical marijuana such as the drug's effects on the body, the illnesses for which it may be suitable, proper administration of the drug, its potential side effects, and legal consequences associated with its use.

Castle, David J., Robin Murray, and Deepak Cyril D'Souza. *Marijuana and Madness*, 2nd ed. Cambridge and New York: Cambridge University Press, 2012.

This book provides a highly technical and detailed review of the existing scientific evidence about the relationship between marijuana use and mental illness.

Caulkins, Jonathan P., Mark A. R. Kleiman, Angela Hawken, and Beau Kilmer. *Marijuana Legalization: What Everyone Needs to Know.* New York: Oxford University Press, 2012.

This book is based on the presumption that individual states in the United States will soon begin passing laws to legalize the use of marijuana for recreational and medical purposes. The authors' objective here is to provide essential background information on this topic, including physical and psychological consequences of marijuana use, current laws and proposed legislation, possible effects of legalizing marijuana at the state and national level, and suggestions for ways in which the drug could be produced and regulated.

Clark, Ethan L., ed. *Cannabis Sativa for Health and Hemp.* New York: Nova Science Publisher, 2011.

This book takes the somewhat unusual direction of analyzing the debate over the legalization of marijuana for medical purposes and a market survey of the uses of and potential for hemp as an agricultural crop.

Decorte, Tom, Gary Potter, and Martin Bouchard. *World Wide Weed: Global Trends in Cannabis Cultivation and its Control.* Farnham, UK: Ashgate, 2011.

The authors provide a technical review of the cultivation of the cannabis plant in many parts of the world with a discussion of the role of illegal markets in the economy of the plant.

Deitch, Robert. *Hemp: American History Revisited: The Plant with a Divided History.* New York: Algora Publishing, 2003.

The author presents a detailed history of the role of cannabis in the United States from the colonial period to the present day. In spite of the book's name, it deals with both hemp and marijuana—their production, use, and legal status.

Earleywine, Mitch. *Understanding Marijuana: A New Look at the Scientific Evidence.* Oxford and New York: Oxford University Press, 2005.

After an introductory chapter on the history of marijuana, the author reviews research dealing with topics such as the drug's impact on thought and memory, the pharmacology of cannabis, marijuana's health effects, the medical uses of marijuana, and law and policy issues.

Emmett, David, and Graeme Nice. *What You Need to Know about Cannabis: Understanding the Facts.* London and Philadelphia: Jessica Kingsley Publishers, 2009.

The authors present a comprehensive, traditional overview of the use of cannabis for recreational and health purposes, with a legal and law enforcement emphasis. They provide chapters on the botany and pharmacology of cannabis, medical uses of the plant, detection of marijuana use, cannabis and the law, and the global cannabis industry.

Fox, Steve, Paul Armentano, and Mason Tvert. *Marijuana Is Safer: So Why Are We Driving People to Drink?* White River Junction, VT: Chelsea Green Publishing, 2009.

The authors focus on the two most commonly used recreational drugs in the world, alcohol and marijuana, one legal and one illegal. Of the two, the health consequences of alcohol are demonstrably more serious than those of marijuana. What are the forces, then, that drive individuals to use alcohol far more commonly than they use marijuana, and what are the societal forces that reinforce that trend?

Geluradi, John. *Cannabiz: The Explosive Rise of the Medical Marijuana Industry.* Sausalito, CA: PoliPoint Press, 2010.

The author discusses the history of the marijuana growing business and how it has grown from a largely counter-cultural activity to a major commercial business in many parts of the world. He considers how legalization of the drug might affect this new agribusiness.

Gerber, Rudolph Joseph. *Legalizing Marijuana: Drug Policy Reform and Prohibition Politics.* Westport, CT: Praeger, 2004.

The author reviews a history of the criminalization of marijuana and then provides an extended argument as to why that criminalization has not worked and why use of the drug should now be decriminalized.

Gross, Frederick C., and Reeve Chace. *The Truth about Marijuana.* New York: Rosen Publishing, 2012.

This book is intended for high school readers. It provides a general background on marijuana, including the physical and psychological effects of ingesting marijuana, drug testing, dependence and withdrawal, and sources for help and treatment.

Grotenhermen, Franjo, and Ethan Russo. *Cannabis and Cannabinoids: Pharmacology, Toxicology, and Therapeutic Potential.* New York: Haworth Integrative Healing Press, 2002.

This is a technical and useful book providing fundamental information on many aspects of the cannabis plant and its chemical analogs.

Herer, Jack. *The Emperor Wears No Clothes,* 11th ed. Anaheim, CA: AH HA Publishing, 2001.

The publisher claims that this book is the "authoritative history of hemp's myriad uses and of the war on this plant." The book certainly contains a wealth of detailed information about the history of the plant, its many uses, and efforts to make its use for recreational purposes illegal. Text of the book is also available online at http://www.hampapartiet.se/25.pdf.

Holland, Julie, ed. *The Pot Book: A Complete Guide to Cannabis: Its Role in Medicine, Politics, Science, and Culture.* Rochester, VT: Park Street Press, 2010.

This book is a superb review of the many aspects of the cannabis debate. Part I deals with a scientific overview of the plant, its chemical composition and biological effects. Part II discusses risk of harm and use reduction. Part III focuses on the clinical uses of marijuana. Part IV deals with the cannabis culture. And Part V concludes with a review of governmental policies and various recommendations that represent steps in "the right direction," according to the editor.

Iversen, Leslie L. *The Science of Marijuana*, 2nd ed. New York and Oxford: Oxford University Press, 2008.

This book discusses the technical aspects of cannabis, including topics such as the biosynthesis and pharmacology of endocannabinoids, the effects of cannabis on the central nervous system, synthetic cannabinoids, and medical uses of cannabis.

Jacquette, Dale, ed. *Cannabis: Philosophy for Everyone: What Were We Just Talking About?* Malden, MA: Wiley-Blackwell, 2010.

This collection of essays deals with a variety of cannabis-related topics, including cannabis phenomenology, marijuana and spiritual enlightenment, effects of cannabis use on creativity, psychosocial dimensions of the cannabis culture, and ethics and politics of cannabis use.

Johnson, Albert T., ed. *Medical Marijuana and Marijuana Use.* New York: Nova Science, 2009.

This short book consists of just two chapters, the first of which outlines the Office of National Drug Control Policy's views on cannabis use. The second and much longer chapter reviews and analyzes policies related to the medical use of marijuana at the federal and various state levels.

Kamin, Sam, and Christopher S. Morris. *The Impact of the Decriminalization and Legalization of Marijuana: An Immediate Look at the Cannabis Reform Movement.* Boston: Aspatore, 2010.

The authors drawn on the expertise of legal scholars throughout the United States to get predictions as to the possible legal, social, political, and other effects resulting from the increasing amount of decriminalization and/or legalization of marijuana use currently taking place in the United States.

Lee, Martin A. *Smoke Signals A Social History of Marijuana: Medical, Recreational & Scientific.* New York: Scribner's, 2012.

Lee discusses the battle between the federal government and proponents of cannabis use beginning in the 1960s and notes the number of ways in whch the latter group has managed to overcome the powerful forces of the federal government to make marijuana a vibrant part of everyday modern life in the United States.

London, Jeffrey Matthew. *How the Use of Marijuana Was Criminalized and Medicalized, 1906–2004: A Foucaultian History of Legislation in America.* Lewiston, NY: Edwin Mellen Press, 2009.

The author provides a scholarly analysis of the process by which marijuana was criminalized during the 20th century. He then describes the process by which medical marijuana developed an increasingly wide audience and general acceptance during the last few decades of the century.

Mack, Alison, and Janet Elizabeth Joy. *Marijuana as Medicine?: The Science beyond the Controversy.* Washington, DC: National Academy Press, 2001.

This book is a report of a study conducted by the U.S. Institute of Medicine on the scientific information available about the medical benefits of marijuana. The report summarizes not only the drug's general medical benefits, but also its potential for harm, legal issues, and marijuana's medical effects on a number of specific diseases, such as HIV/AIDS, cancer, and glaucoma.

Martin, Mickey, and Dale H. Gieringer. *Medical Marijuana 101: Everything They Told You Is Wrong.* Oakland, CA: Quick American Archives, 2012.

The authors attempt to explain why much of the information provided to the general public about the health effects of marijuana is incorrect. They then go on to describe and discuss the growing movement for the medical use of marijuana and the present status of that movement.

McCabe, John. *Hemp: What the World Needs Now.* Santa Monica, CA: Carmania Books, 2010.

This book focuses almost entirely on the uses of hemp and its potential value as a cash crop in the world today. It argues that the use of hemp has been hampered by the "bad press" associated with its cannabis cousin, marijuana.

Merino, Noël. *Medical Marijuana.* Farmington Hills, MI: Greenhaven Press, 2011.

This title, in Greenhaven's Current Controversies series, explores the use of marijuana for medical purposes, including its effectiveness, legal and ethical concerns, and effects of individual state laws on the subject.

Mills, James H. *Cannabis Britannica: Empire, Trade, and Prohibition, 1800–1928.* Oxford and New York: Oxford University Press, 2003.

The author provides a fascinating history of British attitudes toward cannabis and the role of the substance in British history over the time period given.

Mills, James H. *Madness, Cannabis and Colonialism: The "Native Only" Lunatic Asylums of British India, 1857–1900.* London: Palgrave Macmillan, 2000.

The author reports on the creation of lunatic asylums by the British government following the Indian rebellion of 1857 as a way of keeping itinerant natives under control. The asylums were apparently occupied almost exclusively by individuals who had been users of cannabis products.

Nores, John, and James A. Swan. *War in the Woods: Combating Marijuana Cartels on America's Public Lands.* Guilford, CT: Lyons Press, 2010.

The authors, a warden for the California Fish and Game Commission and a columnist for ESPN, describe episodes that have occurred during efforts to find and destroy marijuana crops on public lands. They discuss the threat to human life and the environmental damage caused by illegal marijuana farms.

Oner, S. T., ed. *Cannabis Indica: The Essential Guide to the World's Finest Marijuana Strains.* San Francisco: Green Candy Press, 2011.

See annotation under following title.

Oner, S. T., ed. *Cannabis Sativa: The Essential Guide to the World's Finest Marijuana Strains.* San Francisco: Green Candy Press, 2012.

These two books provide perhaps the most exhaustive review of the two most widely used species of cannabis among individuals who use marijuana as a recreational drug. The authors provide very detailed reviews of more than 100 different strains of each species, including background on their genetic development, potency, and source of seeds.

Pennsylvania Bar Institute. *Legalizing Marijuana.* Mechanicsburg: Pennsylvania Bar Institute, 2011.

This publication reviews the legal status of both marijuana in general and medical marijuana in particular, with chapters on federal policy on the topics, state actions on medical marijuana, and proposed Pennsylvania legislation on the topic.

Regan, Trish. *Joint Ventures: Inside America's Almost Legal Marijuana Industry.* Hoboken, NJ: Wiley, 2011.

This book provides a detailed look at the business of growing and marketing marijuana in the United States, with consideration of how legalization might affect the marijuana market.

Robinson, Rowan. *The Great Book of Hemp: The Complete Guide to the Environmental, Commercial, and Medicinal Uses of the World's Most Extraordinary Plant.* Rochester, VT: Park Street Press, 1996.

This book provides an excellent history of the role of hemp in human civilization, with a good introduction to social and economic issues associated with its use in the past and currently.

Rojas, Andrea S., ed. *Marijuana: Uses, Effects and the Law.* New York: Nova Science, 2011.

This book focuses on issues related to the medical use of marijuana such as problems involved in determining the amount of cannabis delivered by various types of treatment, the effect of marijuana legislation on vulnerable populations, the physical and psychological effects of marijuana, and the use of marijuana by adolescents.

Room, Robin et al. *Cannabis Policy: Moving beyond Stalemate.* Oxford: Oxford University Press, 2010.

This book reviews the findings of a conference sponsored by the Beckley Foundation on marijuana policy around the world. Part I of this book provides an overview of the existing state of marijuana policy, with attention to the effects of marijuana use, current market and legal policies, and some steps that can be taken to get beyond the current impasse over marijuana policy. Part II discusses recommendations of the Cannabis Convention, and Part III provides a draft framework convention on a new approach to marijuana policy.

Rubin, Vera D., ed. *Cannabis and Culture.* The Hague: Mouton, 1975.

This book includes papers presented at the Ninth International Congress of the International Union of Anthropological and Ethnological Sciences held in Chicago in 1973. It contains fascinating articles on a range of cannabis-related topics, including "Early Diffusion and Folk Uses of Hemp," "The Origin and Use of Cannabis in Eastern Asia: Their Linguistic-Cultural Implications," "The Social Nexus of Ganja in Jamaica," "The Ritual Use of Cannabis in Mexico," "Traditional Patterns of Hashish Use in Egypt," "Social and Medical Aspects of the Use of Cannabis in Brazil," "Sociocultural and Epidemiological Aspects of Hashish Use in Greece," "Memories, Reflections and Myths: The American Marihuana Commission," and "Sociocultural Factors in Marihuana Use in the United States."

Russo, Ethan, and Franjo Grotenhermen, eds. *Handbook of Cannabis Therapeutics: From Bench to Bedside.* New York: Haworth Press, 2006.

This book is divided into five major sections dealing with historical notes, pharmacology and pharmacokinetics, endocannabinoids and cannabinoid receptors, and side effects. It is a valuable resource on most of the fundamental issues related to the medical uses of marijuana.

Stolick, Matthew. *Otherwise Law-Abiding Citizens: A Scientific and Moral Assessment of Cannabis Use.* Lanham, MD: Lexington Books, 2009.

The author draws on the writings of noted philosophers to develop a moral analysis of the use of marijuana as a recreational drug. He shows how both scientific information and moral concepts have led to current legal and political positions on the use of marijuana.

Wilson, Hugh T. *Annual Editions: Drugs, Society, and Behavior 2011/2012*, 26th ed. Boston: McGraw-Hill Higher Education, 2012.

Annual Editions is regularly updated to provide expert views on the most important social topics of the day. Each book, written for the layperson, contains articles from newspapers, magazines, and journals written by experts in the field. The book comes with a resource guide and relevant testing materials.

Periodicals

Abrams, D. I. et al. 2007. "Cannabis in Painful HIV-Associated Sensory Neuropathy: A Randomized Placebo-Controlled Trial." *Neurology* 68(7): 515–521.

The research team finds that smoked marijuana is as effective as standard medications for the reduction of pain associated with HIV/AIDS-related neuropathy. Reviewers of the research note that "[i]t is a sad commentary on the state of modern medicine that we still need 'proof' of something that medicine has known for 5,000 years."

Acworth, Alex, Nicolas de Roos, and Hajime Katayama. 2012. "Substance Use and Adolescent Sexual Activity." *Applied Economics* 44(9): 1067–1079.

The authors explore the relationship between early drug use and initiation of sexual activity among adolescents and find a strong correlation between the two for males, but no correlation for females.

Andresen, Stina Troldtoft, and Sabine Karg. 2011. "Retting Pits for Textile Fibre Plants at Danish Prehistoric Sites Dated

Between 800 B.C. and A.D. 1050." *Vegetation History and Archaeobotany* 20(6): 517–526.

The authors report on recent archaeological finds of relatively sophisticated methods ("retting") for separating hemp fibers from the cannabis plant at a period in Europe much earlier than had previously been thought.

Bonnie, Richard J., and Charles H. Whitebread. 1970. "The Forbidden Fruit and the Tree of Knowledge: An Inquiry into the Legal History of American Marijuana Prohibition." *Virginia Law Review* 56(6): 971–1203.

This article is the basis for a book written by Bonnie and Whitebread on the history of the criminalization of cannabis in the United States (see "Books" earlier in this chapter). It is widely regarded as one of the most (if not *the* most) complete reports and analyses of this story. It is also available in full online at http://www.druglibrary.org/schaffer/LIBRARY/studies/vlr/vlrtoc.htm.

Brunner, Theodore F. 1973. "Marijuana in Ancient Greece and Rome? The Literary Evidence." *Bulletin of the History of Medicine* 47(4): 344–355.

The author uses literary sources to make his case that the Greeks and Romans were familiar with the medical uses of cannabis and included it in their materia medica, but that there is no evidence that they knew of or took advantage of its psychoactive effects.

Campos, Isaac. 2010. "Degeneration and the Origins of Mexico's War on Drugs." *Mexican Studies/Estudios Mexicanos* 26(2): 379–408.

The author traces the events that led to the initiation of the war against drugs in Mexico, beginning with a constitutional provision making marijuana and other drugs illegal in 1917 and then continuing with an aggressive war on drugs beginning in 1920.

Cerda, Magdalena et al. 2012. "Medical Marijuana Laws in 50 States: Investigating the Relationship between State Legalization of Medical Marijuana and Marijuana Use, Abuse and Dependence." *Drug and Alcohol Dependence* 120(1–3): 22–27.

Researchers found that the rate of marijuana use was higher in states that have medical marijuana laws than those that do not.

De Vries, I., C. Hunault, A. Van Riel, and J. Meulenbelt. 2010. "Cannabis Acute and Chronic Effects: The Dutch Experience." *Toxicology Letters* 196: S15.

Reflecting a difference in Dutch policy on cannabis use from that of nearly all other nations, a regular effort is made to assess the effects of marijuana use within the Dutch population. This summary says that the "acute toxicity of cannabis is low," there is a large variability in acute effects among users, cannabis can contribute to the onset of mental problems among individuals who are already at risk for such problems, and there is a slight risk for increased likelihood of depression.

Di Marzo, V., and F. Piscitelli. 2011. "Gut Feelings about the Endocannabinoid System." *Neurogastroenterology & Motility* 23(5): 391–398.

This article provides a technical and detailed description of the role and function of the endocannabinoid system in the gastrointestinal system.

DiNitto, Diana M., and Namkee G. Choi. 2011. "Marijuana Use among Older Adults in the U.S.A.: User Characteristics, Patterns of Use, and Implications for Intervention." *International Psychogeriatrics* 23(5): 732–741.

The authors point out that the use of marijuana is increasing among older individuals, especially among those in the "younger range of the older population." They recommend that social service workers become more aware of this trend and be prepared to offer marijuana users assistance in dealing with psychological problems associated with this pattern of behavior.

D'Souza, Deepak Cyril, Richard Andrew Sewell, and Mohini Ranganathan. 2009. "Cannabis and Psychosis/Schizophrenia: Human Studies." *European Archives of Psychiatry and Clinical Neuroscience* 7: 413–431.

The authors discuss some of the mechanisms by which cannabinoids may affect the human nervous system, causing the development of psychoses and/or schizophrenia. They conclude that the substance may be implicated in the development of mental disorders but only in "a very small proportion of the general population."

Du Toit, Brian M. 1996. "Pot by Any Other Name Is Still . . . A Study of the Diffusion of Cannabis." *South African Journal of Ethnology* 19(4): 127–135.

This paper traces the diffusion of the cannabis plant through (mostly northern) Africa and into Europe, with special attention to the various names by which the plant was known and the uses to which it was put.

Dyer, Owen. 2008. "Government Tightens Rules on Cannabis Despite Recommendation Not to Do So." *BMJ* 336(7653): 1095. Also available online at http://www.ncbi.nlm.nih.gov/pmc/articles/PMC2386588/.

The Home Secretary of the United Kingdom announces that the government will reclassify marijuana from a class C drug to a class B drug, increasing penalties for possession from two to five years, even though the advisory committee on the issue voted 20 to three against such a reclassification.

Farrimond, Jonathan A. et al. 2011. "*Cannabis sativa* and the Endogenous Cannabinoid System: Therapeutic Potential for Appetite Regulation." *Phytotherapy Research* 25(2): 170–188.

The authors review the endocannabinoid system as well as its response to THC and its analogs and come to the conclusion that "non-Δ^9-tetrahydrocannabinol phytocannabinoids retain an important and, as yet, untapped clinical potential."

Fernández-Artamendi, Sergio, José R. Fernández-Hermida, Roberto Secades-Villa, and Paz García-Portilla. 2011. "Cannabis and Mental Health." *Actas Españolas De Psiquiatría* 39(3): 180–190.

The authors review nearly 100 research studies dealing with marijuana and mental health, and find no causality relationship between marijuana use and mental disorder, although they also conclude that "a risk for mental health seems to exist for regular users with a certain vulnerability or predisposition, in whom cannabis use significantly increases the risks of presenting mental disorders, particularly psychotic disorders."

Hall, Waynea, and Michaelb Lynskey. 2009. "The Challenges in Developing a Rational Cannabis Policy." *Current Opinion in Psychiatry* 22(3): 258–262.

The authors point out and analyze the major conflict in developing a rational cannabis policy, the desire on the one hand to prevent users from being exposed to a substance that has been implicated in a variety of physical, mental, and emotional disorders and, on the other hand, avoiding the huge investment of time, money, and personnel needed to maintain the current ban on cannabis.

Järvinen, Margaretha, and Jeanette Østergaard. 2011. "Dangers and Pleasures: Drug Attitudes and Experiences among Young People." *Acta Sociologica* 54(4): 333–350.

The authors report on a study of 17- to 19-year-old Danes that sought to determine their attitudes toward drugs and drinking, reported drug use by friends, and their own experiences with drug use. They identify four general attitudes about drug use, which they classify as anti-drug, ambivalent, transitory, and pro-drug.

Kalant, Harold. 2001. "Medicinal Use of Cannabis: History and Current Status." *Pain Research and Management* 6(Part II): 80–94.

The author reviews the history of the use of cannabis products for therapeutic purposes, as well as recent developments in the field. He comes to the conclusion that the substance has valid and useful therapeutic applications, although the use of the drug or its components orally, rectally, or parenterally would probably result in fewer side effects than would smoking. He predicts that future research may produce marijuana analogs that are even safer to use than existing natural products.

Kalant, Oriana Josseau. 1971. "Ludlow on Cannabis: A Modern Look at a Nineteenth Century Drug Experience." *International Journal of the Addictions* 6(2): 309–322. Also available online at http://druglibrary.net/schaffer/History/kalant.htm.

One of the most famous books in the history of cannabis studies is *The Hasheesh Eater*, written by American Fitz Hugh Ludlow in 1857. In this book, Ludlow describes in detail his experiences as a user of hashish over many years. This article analyzes some of the important information to be gained about hashish from that book.

Kendell, Robert. 2003. "Cannabis Condemned: The Proscription of Indian Hemp." *Addiction* (Abingdon, England) 98(2): 143–151.

The author provides some interesting history about the process by which marijuana became criminalized internationally, beginning with a 1925 League of Nations conference on opium, at which marijuana was declared by Egyptian representatives to represent a threat as serious as that posed by opium.

Kozma, Liat. 2011. "Cannabis Prohibition in Egypt, 1880–1939: From Local Ban to League of Nations Diplomacy." *Middle Eastern Studies* 47(2): 443–460.

This article is a valuable antidote to the general historical view that international antidrug policies in the second half of the 20th century grew out of the proliferation of U.S. antidrug policies. The author demonstrates that many countries around the world were instrumental in developing their own and international laws to deal with illegal substances.

Kozma, Liat. 2011. "The League of Nations and the Debate over Cannabis Prohibition." *History Compass* 9(1): 61–70.

The author explores the work of a subcommittee largely responsible for the development of League policies on cannabis use and transport. He points out that the positions eventually taken by the League reflected certain colonial assumptions about Arabs and Muslims.

Lu, Xiaozhai, and Robert C. Clarke. 1995. "The Cultivation and Use of Hemp *(Cannabis Sativa L.)* in Ancient China." *Journal of the International Hemp Association* 2(1):26–30. Archived online at http://www.internationalhempassociation .org/jiha/iha02111.html.

This article provides an excellent detailed review of the early use of cannabis for a variety of purposes in ancient China.

Lucas, Philippe. 2009. "Moral Regulation and the Presumption of Guilt in Health Canada's Medical Cannabis Policy and Practice." *International Journal of Drug Policy* 20(4): 296–303.

The Canadian government provides therapeutic marijuana to patients through Health Canada's Marihuana Medical Access Division (MMAD). The program assumes, the author says, that applicants for the program have other than medical reasons for applying and that they are viewed, therefore, as being "inherently guilty." He points out that this bias on the part of the federal agency prevents it from achieving its goals of providing for individuals who would truly benefit from therapeutic marijuana, and that certain community-based medical marijuana programs are far more effective in achieving this objective.

Macleod, J., and M. Hickman. 2010. "How Ideology Shapes the Evidence and the Policy: What Do We Know about Cannabis Use and What Should We Do?" *Addiction* 105(8): 1326–1330.

The authors point out that in most countries, the use of marijuana is usually considered in the context of criminology rather than public health. They suggest that this approach may not be the best way of dealing with both the personal health and social issues associated with cannabis use.

McCrystal, Patrick, and Kerry Winning. 2009. "Cannabis Reclassification: What Is the Message to the Next Generation of Cannabis Users?" *Child Care in Practice* 15(1): 57–73.

The authors ask how the British government's downgrading cannabis from a class B to a class C substance has affected the way young people in Great Britain view use of the drug. They conclude that it is too early to say but express their own bias that the government action may allow young people to know less or feel less concerned about possible negative consequences of cannabis use.

Merlin, M. D. 2003. "Archaeological Evidence for the Tradition of Psychoactive Plant Use in the Old World." *Economic Botany* 57(3): 295–323.

The author provides an extensive and detailed review of the ways in which psychoactive drugs, including marijuana, were used for a variety of purposes perhaps as far back as 12,000 years ago.

Mikuriya, Tod H. 1969. "Marijuana in Medicine: Past, Present and Future." *California Medicine* 110(1): 34–40. Also available online at http://www.ncbi.nlm.nih.gov/pmc/articles/PMC1503422/pdf/califmed00019-0036.pdf.

This article is of historic importance because it was written by the most outspoken advocate of medical marijuana within the medical profession long before it became a topic of general interest in the late 20th century.

Monshouwer, Karin, Margriet Van Laar, and Wilma A. Vollebergh. 2011. "Buying Cannabis in 'Coffee Shops.'" *Drug and Alcohol Review* 30(2): 148–156.

For some time, the sale of cannabis products in Dutch coffee shops has been legal. This study suggests that the amount of substance abuse in the Netherlands is generally less than in the rest of Europe, although somewhat higher than average among adolescents. The public availability of marijuana does not appear to have increased problems of substance abuse in Holland.

Morningstar, Patricia J. 1985. "Thandai and Chilam: Traditional Hindu Beliefs about the Proper Uses of Cannabis." *Journal of Psychoactive Drugs* 17(3): 141–165.

The author points out that cannabis has some diverse and contradictory effects on the human body, which may make it difficult for a society to know how to classify use of the substance. She demonstrates how traditional Indian culture has resolved this problem over centuries of use of the drug for a variety of purposes, always taking advantage of its benefits while placing acknowledging and attempting to reduce its potential risks.

Nahas, Gabriel G. 1982. "Hashish in Islam: 9th to 18th Century." *Bulletin of the New York Academy of Medicine* 58(9): 814–831. Also available online at http://www.ncbi.nlm.nih.gov/pmc/articles/PMC1805385/pdf/bullnyacadmed00095-0056.pdf.

The author offers a superb review of the use of hashish in the Muslim Middle East during the time period mentioned in the article title.

Pedersen, Willy, and Torbjørn Skardhamar. 2009. "Cannabis and Crime: Findings from a Longitudinal Study." *Addiction* 105(1): 109–118.

The authors follow 1,353 individuals from the Young in Norway Longitudinal Study (between the ages of 13 and 27) and find that those who smoke marijuana as youngsters are more likely to be associated with criminal activities in their adult years, although those activities are generally restricted to drug-related crimes. Also see the response to this article, Bretteville-Jensen, Anne Line, and Ingeborg Rossow. 2010. "Questionable Conclusions on Cannabis and Crime." *Addiction* 106(2): 449–450

Reece, Albert Stuart. 2009. "Chronic Toxicology of Cannabis." *Clinical Toxicology* 47(6): 517–524.

The author reviewed 5,198 scientific papers on the chronic toxicology of cannabis and came to the conclusion that chronic cannabis use is associated with psychiatric, respiratory, cardiovascular, and bone effects as well as oncogenic, teratogenic, and mutagenic effects. All of these effects depend on dose and duration of use.

Reinarman, Craig, Peter D. A. Cohen, and Hendrien L. Kaal. 2004. "The Limited Relevance of Drug Policy: Cannabis in Amsterdam and in San Francisco." *American Journal of Public Health* 94(5): 836–842. Also available online at http://www.mapinc.org/lib/limited.pdf.

The authors test the hypothesis that punishment for cannabis use deters use and thereby benefits public health and find that the hypothesis does not hold. They conclude that "experienced users . . . appear to regulate their cannabis use so as to minimize the risk that it will interfere with normal social functioning."

Rongione, Danielle, Bradley Erford, and Caren Broglie. 2011. "Alcohol and Other Drug Abuse Counseling Outcomes for School-Aged Youth: A Meta-Analysis of Studies from 1990 to 2009." *Counseling Outcome Research and Evaluation* 2(1): 8–24.

In their review of 20 studies consisting of 2,837 participants, the authors found "no substantial effects of moderating variables."

Russo, Ethan. 2002. "Cannabis Treatments in Obstetrics and Gynecology: A Historical Review." *Journal of Cannabis Therapeutics* 2(3–4): 5–34. Also available online at http://www.freedomtoexhale.com/russo-ob.pdf.

The author points out that there is a long history associated with the use of cannabis for a variety of obstetrical and gynecological problems. He concludes from his own studies that cannabis may have useful applications in dealing with a variety of female disorders including dysmenorrhea, dysuria, hyperemesis gravidarum, and menopausal symptoms.

Russo, Ethan et al. 2002. "Chronic Cannabis Use in the Compassionate Investigational New Drug Program: An Examination of Benefits and Adverse Effects of Legal Clinical Cannabis." *Journal of Cannabis Therapeutics* 2(1): 3–57. Also available online at http://www.maps.org/mmj/russo2002.pdf.

The U.S. government has operated an Investigational New Drug program for the compassionate use of marijuana for the treatment of certain severe medical disorders since 1976. At the time of this study, eight people remained in the program. The authors attempted to determine the effects on these individuals of almost 30 years of smoking low-grade (i.e., low-concentration of THC) marijuana. They found that patients experienced relief from the most serious of their medical problems accompanied by no significant physical, medical, emotional, or other problems. They recommended that the Investigational New Drug program be reopened for individuals who can benefit from cannabis therapy.

Saper, Anthony. 1974. "The Making of Policy through Myth, Fantasy and Historical Accident: the Making of America's Narcotics Laws." *British Journal of Addiction to Alcohol and Other Drugs* 69(2): 183–193.

The author agues that drug laws in the United States during the first three quarters of the 20th century were made on the basis of "myth, fantasy, historical accident; interwoven with occasional rationality."

Schubart, C. D. et al. 2011. "Association between Cannabis and Psychiatric Hospitalization." *Acta Psychiatrica Scandinavica* 123 (5): 368–375.

Based on an analysis of 17,698 individuals with a history of hospitalization for psychiatric problems, the authors conclude that "early and heavy uses of cannabis are each and independently associated with poor mental health in its users."

Shamloul, Rany, and Anthony J. Bella. 2011. "Impact of Cannabis Use on Male Sexual Health." *Journal of Sexual Medicine* 8(4): 971–975.

The authors review the available scientific evidence on the topic posed in the title of the article and find that the results of such research are ambiguous and contradictory, leaving us not yet knowing the answer to the question.

Small, Ernest, and Arthur Cronquist. 1976. "Practical and Natural Taxonomy for Cannabis." *Taxon* 25(4): 405–435.

This paper is of special, if somewhat dated, interest in the question of the taxonomic status of the various forms of cannabis.

Temple, E. C., R. F. Brown, and D. W. Hine. 2011. "The 'Grass Ceiling': Limitations in the Literature Hinder Our

Understanding of Cannabis Use and Its Consequences." *Addiction* 106(2): 238–244.

The authors discuss methodological problems that limit the usefulness of the vast amount of research that has been done on cannabis use. Of special interest is a response to these articles: Earleywine, Mitch. "The Elephant in the Room with the 'Grass Ceiling.' " *Addiction* 106(2): 245–246; and Copeland, Jan. "The Glass Ceiling on Evidence of Cannabis Related Harms: Flawed or Just False?" *Addiction* 106(2): 249–251.

Touw, Mia. 1981. "The Religious and Medicinal Uses of Cannabis in China, India and Tibet." *Journal of Psychoactive Drugs* 13(1): 23–34. Also available online at http://www.cnsproductions.com/pdf/Touw.pdf.

The author provides a somewhat abbreviated but interesting review of the ways in which cannabis was used in the early history of East Asia.

Vandrey, R., K. E. Dunn, J. A. Fry, and E. R. Girling. 2012. "A Survey Study to Characterize Use of Spice Products (Synthetic Cannabinoids)." *Drug and Alcohol Dependence* 120(1–3): 238–241.

Spice is the name given to a relatively new drug consisting of natural herbs treated with synthetic cannabinoids. Little research has been done on the use of the drug, which is illegal in most parts of the world. The authors found that most users continued to seek access to the drug even after it had been declared illegal.

Van Gundy, Karen, and Cesar Rebellon. 2010. "A Life-Course Perspective on the 'Gateway Hypothesis.' " *Journal of Health and Social Behavior* 51(3): 244–259.

The researchers investigate the common belief among drug researchers and policymakers that marijuana is a "gateway" drug, that is, one that leads to increased risk for other forms of substance abuse later in life. They conclude that in the most general terms, the hypothesis may be correct, but confounding factors make the relationship much more complex. For example, they discover a low correlation between early marijuana use and later substance abuse among those who are employed early in life. They also find that the conversion from marijuana to other drugs is often short lived, and that users often discontinue substance abuse quite early in life.

Van Ours, Jan C. and Jenny Williams. 2011. "Cannabis Use and Mental Health Problems." *Journal of Applied Econometrics* 26(7): 1137–1156.

The authors investigate the hypothesis that early marijuana use may lead to later mental health problems but find that current use is a more important predictor of mental health problems than is early use, and that the amount of marijuana used is strongly related to possible mental health problems.

Weinstein, A. M., and David A. Gorelick. 2011. "Pharmacological Treatment of Cannabis Dependence." *Current Pharmaceutical Design* 17(14): 1351–1358.

The authors discuss the need for drugs for the treatment of marijuana addiction, withdrawal symptoms and related problems, the current unavailability of such drugs, and some promising candidate substances for treatment.

Wright, Stephen. 2007. "Cannabinoid-Based Medicines for Neurological Disorders: Clinical Evidence." *Molecular Neurobiology* 36 (1): 129–136.

The author reviews the history of the development of synthetic cannabinoids and the evidence of their therapeutic value, especially in comparison with natural cannabinoids. He concludes that "oral administration of cannabinoids may not be the preferred route of administration and that plant extracts show greater evidence of efficacy than synthetic compounds."

Reports

Broad Public Support For Legalizing Medical Marijuana. Pew Research Center for the People & the Press. http://pewresearch.org/pubs/1548/broad-public-support-for-legalizing-medical-marijuana. Accessed on December 4, 2011.

The polling results reported here suggest that 73 percent of respondents favor legalizing medical marijuana, while 23 percent oppose the practice. The greatest difference among respondents was found between Republicans and Democrats, a difference of about 20 percentage points.

Franco, Celinda. *Federal Domestic Illegal Drug Enforcement Efforts: Are They Working?* Washington, DC: Congressional Research Service, January 2010.

Congress asked the Congressional Research Service (CRS) to assess the effectiveness of the nation's efforts to reduce illegal drug use. The CRS report points out that efforts to solve this problem have not changed since the mid-1980s, although the nature of the nation's "drug problem" has changed significantly over that period of time. The report concludes that there is not enough good research evidence on which to answer the original question, although overall, the nation's drug problem does not appear to have improved much in spite of the time, money, personnel, and other efforts expended to reduce substance abuse.

Life Sentences: Collateral Sanctions Associated with Marijuana Offenses. Center for Cognitive Liberty & Ethics. http://www.cognitiveliberty.org/rpts/col_sanctions.htm. Accessed on December 12, 2011.

This report is based on the assumption that a prison or jail sentence and/or fine for possession of marijuana is not the total sanction imposed for the crime. Instead, a person may experience socially and personally destructive consequences as the result of such a conviction, including loss of the right to adopt a child, loss of the eligibility to be a foster parent, loss of the right to vote, and loss of the right to serve on a jury. The report lists these additional sanctions for each state and ranks the states in this regard from severe to moderate.

Marijuana Abuse. Washington, DC: National Institute on Drug Abuse, October 2002; revised September 2010.

This publication claims to provide the latest reliable scientific information on the effect of marijuana use on animals.

Ramström, Jan. *Adverse Health Consequences of Cannabis Use: A Survey of Scientific Studies Published up to and Including 2008.* Östersund: Swedish National Institute of Public Health, 2009.

This report provides a thorough review of research done on the physical, mental, psychosocial, and psychological effects of marijuana use.

Results from the 2010 National Survey on Drug Use and Health: Summary of National Findings. Rockville, MD: U.S. Department of Health and Human Services. Substance Abuse and Mental Health Services Administration. Center for Behavioral Health Statistics and Quality, September 2011. Also available online at http://www.samhsa.gov/data/NSDUH/2k10NSDU H/2k10Results.htm.

This report is issued annually and provides complete statistical data on the use of legal and illegal drugs by individuals of all ages, both genders, and all ethnic backgrounds in the United States.

Spicer, Leah. *Historical and Cultural Uses of Cannabis and the Canadian "Marijuana Clash."* Report prepared for the Senate Special Committee On Illegal Drugs. http://www.parl.gc.ca/

Content/SEN/Committee/371/ille/library/spicer-e.htm#2. Central Asia. Accessed on December 18, 2011.

This report was prepared to give background information on the history of cannabis use for a Canadian committee studying possible changes in policy for that nation in 2002. It is a complete and detailed description of the history of cannabis use from the earliest days of human civilization.

The State of the Drugs Problem in Europe. European Monitoring Centre for Drugs and Drug Abuse. Luxembourg: Publications Office of the European Union, 2010. Also available online at http://www.emcdda.europa.eu/attachements.cfm/att_120104 _EN_EMCDDA_AR2010_EN.pdf.

This annual report provides a broad and detailed summary of the status of substance abuse within the 27 nations that make up the European Union. The publication is an essential up-to-date guide of statistical data and analysis on the issue.

U.S. Department of Justice. National Drug Intelligence Center. *National Drug Threat Assessment.* [n.p.] August 2011. Also available online at http://www.justice.gov/ndic/pubs44/44849/ 44849p.pdf.

This annual publication is published for the purpose of providing policymakers and counterdrug executives with information about the potential threat from drugs as well as from gangs and violence associated with drug use. The 2011 report, for example, focused on the impact of drug use on productivity, crime and criminal systems, and health and health care systems; on transnational criminal organizations; drug trafficking and drug smuggling; drug movement and drug use in the United States; and abuse of prescription drugs.

White House. *National Drug Control Strategy.* http://www .whitehouse.gov/sites/default/files/ondcp/ndcs2011.pdf. Accessed on December 5, 2011.

The president of the United States annually sends Congress a report on the current status of drug use in the United States and federal plans for dealing with that problem in the coming year. The 2011 report is provided here.

World Drug Report 2011. [n.p.]: UN Office on Drug and Crime, 2011.

This extremely valuable report is issued annually, providing an overview of the use of drugs throughout the world. The report provides comprehensive and useful statistics on the production, trafficking, and consumption of cannabis, cocaine, heroin, morphine, and amphetamine-type substances on a worldwide, regional, and national basis. Chapter 5 provides a comprehensive and detailed discussion of the cannabis market.

Nonprint Resources

"100 Peer-Reviewed Studies on Marijuana." ProCon.org. http://medicalmarijuana.procon.org/view.resource.php?resource ID=000884. Accessed on December 8, 2011.

This excellent resource lists 100 scientific studies on marijuana conducted between 1990 and 2011, providing a description of each study, its journal reference, and whether the report produced results in favor of or opposed to the use of marijuana for medical purposes.

Aydin, Ani. "Cannabinoid Poisoning." Medscape Reference. http://emedicine.medscape.com/article/833828-overview. Accessed on January 7, 2012.

This website provides a technical review of the physical, psychological, and other effects of cannabinoids on the human body.

Blanchard, Sean, and Matthew J. Atha. "Indian Hemp and the Dope Fiends of Old England." UKCIA.org. http://www.ukcia. org/culture/history/colonial.php. Accessed on January 7, 2012.

The authors provide an interesting sociopolitical history of cannabis in the British Empire between 1840 and 1928.

Brown, Jeff. "Marijuana and the Bible." http://www.erowid.org/ plants/cannabis/cannabis_spirit2.shtml. Accessed on December 4, 2011.

At the time this work was written, the author was a member of the Ethiopian Zion Coptic Church, which used marijuana as part of its sacraments. The church no longer exists, but the work is of considerable interest in that it attempts to show references in the Bible that apparently refer to the use of marijuana as a psychotropic substance. The work is also available in Kindle edition.

"Cannabis." BBC Health. http://www.bbc.co.uk/health/emotional _health/addictions/cannabis.shtml. Accessed on January 7, 2012.

This site provides a relatively balanced overview of cannabis, its legal status, and its health effects.

"Cannabis." European Monitoring Centre for Drugs and Drug Addiction (EMCDDA). http://www.emcdda.europa.eu/publications/ drug-profiles/cannabis. Accessed on January 7, 2012.

This fact sheet is one of a series published by EMCDDA on various illegal substances. It covers a wide range of topics related to cannabis.

"Cannabis." Vaults of Erowid. http://www.erowid.org/plants/ cannabis/cannabis.shtml. Accessed on January 7, 2012.

The Vaults of Erowid are one of the most extensive and useful sources of information on all aspects of substance use and abuse issues. This website has a large collection of essays on all aspects of cannabis, including botanical information, history of use, drug tests, medical marijuana, and hashish.

"Cannabis and Cannabinoids (PDQ®)." http://cancer.gov/ cancertopics/pdq/cam/cannabis/patient/page1. Accessed on December 4, 2011.

This website is administered by the National Cancer Institute. Therefore, the site focuses on possible medical effects of cannabis and cannabinoids.

"A Cannabis Chronology." UKCIA.org. http://www.ukcia.org/ culture/history/chrono.php. Accessed on December 3, 2011. This website has one of the most complete and detailed Internet histories of cannabis.

"Cannabis/Marijuana (also Hash, Hash Oil and Hemp)." Health Canada. http://www.hc-sc.gc.ca/hc-ps/drugs-drogues/learn-renseigne/ cannabis-eng.php. Accessed on January 7, 2012. This site is a part of Health Canada's series of informational resources on a variety of health issues. It discusses risks and benefits of using marijuana as a recreational drug, as well as a therapeutic agent for various medical disorders.

"Cannabis and Mental Health." Royal College of Psychiatrists. http://www.rcpsych.ac.uk/mentalhealthinfo/problems/alcohol anddrugs/cannabis.aspx. Accessed on January 7, 2012. This useful website contains a great deal of information on possible mental effects of using cannabis, along with a discussion of its current legal status in the United Kingdom. In general, the discussion is based on the assumption that the use of cannabis for recreational purposes is dangerous and generally a bad idea.

"Cannabis News." http://cannabisnews.com/. Accessed on January 7, 2012. This website is hosted by DrugSense MAP, Inc., about which relatively little information is available on the Internet. The website offers recent news on issues related to the decriminalization and legalization of marijuana.

"*Cannabis sativa.*" Flora of North America. http://www.efloras. org/florataxon.aspx?flora_id=1&taxon_id=200006342. Accessed on December 5, 2011.

This website provides a technical description of the cannabis plant.

"The Complete History of Cannabis in Canada." http://www.hackcanada.com/canadian/freedom/hempinfodoc2.html. Accessed on January 7, 2012.

This website reviews important events in the Canadian history of cannabis production and use, along with a legal history of the substance.

Ehrensing, Daryl T. "Feasibility of Industrial Hemp Production in the United States Pacific Northwest." Oregon State University Extension Service. http://extension.oregonstate.edu/catalog/html/sb/sb681/#Economic Importance: Accessed on December 16, 2011.

This website provides one of the most complete and detailed descriptions of the botany and economics of the hemp plant.

"Emerging Clinical Applications for Cannabis and Cannabinoids: A Review of the Recent Scientific Literature, 2000–2010." NORML. http://norml.org/pdf_files/NORML_Clinical_Applications_for_Cannabis_and_Cannabinoids.pdf. Accessed on January 4, 2012.

This report summarizes recent research reports on the use of cannabis and cannabinoids for a wide variety of medical conditions.

Fairy, Bud. "How Marijuana Became Illegal." http://www.ozarkia.net/bill/pot/blunderof37.html. Accessed on December 4, 2011.

This website provides a brief summary of the events that led to the U.S. government's listing marijuana as an illegal substance.

Genen, Lawrence. "Cannabis Compound Abuse." Medscape Reference. http://emedicine.medscape.com/article/286661-overview#showall. Accessed on December 4, 2011.

This website provides detailed information on the medical and psychiatric aspects of marijuana use with sections on pathophysiology, epidemiology, clinical presentation, physical signs and symptoms, causes, differential diagnosis, workup, treatment and management, consultation, medications, outpatient care, deterrence and prevention, complications, prognosis, and patient education.

Gibson, Arthur C. "The Weed of Controversy." http://www.botgard.ucla.edu/html/botanytextbooks/economicbotany/Cannabis/index.html. Accessed on December 4, 2011.

This essay is part of a series on economic botany produced by Gibson, who taught a course on plants and civilization at University of California–Los Angeles (UCLA) for many years. It provides an excellent general introduction to the history of cannabis in human civilization.

Grinspoon, Lester. "History of Cannabis as a Medicine." http://www.maps.org/mmj/grinspoon_history_cannabis_medicine.pdf. Accessed on January 7, 2012.

This statement was prepared for a 2005 legal case in which a patient was suing the Drug Enforcement Administration (DEA) for not allowing him to use marijuana for the treatment of a medical condition.

Guither, Peter. "Why Is Marijuana Illegal?" DrugWarRant.org. http://www.drugwarrant.com/articles/why-is-marijuana-illegal/. Accessed on January 7, 2012.

The author provides an interesting history of the process by which the U.S. government (and other governments) pushed for the criminalization of marijuana during the early part of the 20th century.

"The Health Effects of Marijuana." About.com. http://alcoholism.about.com/od/pot/a/effects.-Lya.htm. Accessed on January 7, 2012.

The effects of marijuana on the brain, heart, and lungs are discussed along with other health issues related to the use of marijuana.

"The History of Medical Cannabis." Antique Cannabis Book. http://antiquecannabisbook.com/chap2B/History.htm. Accessed on January 7, 2012.

This website provides one of the most complete and detailed Internet history of the use of cannabis for medical purposes.

"How Cannabis Was Criminalized." Independent Drug Monitoring Unit. http://www.idmu.co.uk/historical.htm. Accessed on January 7, 2012.

This website provides a detailed history of the events involved in the criminalization of cannabis use in the United Kingdom, beginning with the adoption of the Dangerous Drugs Acts in 1928.

"How Does Marijuana Affect Your Body? What Are the Marijuana Physical Effects? [sic]" Web4Health. http://web4health.info/it/add-cannabis-physical.htm. Accessed on January 7, 2012.

This website provides expert answers to a variety of specific questions about various aspects of cannabis use.

"How Medical Marijuana Works." How Stuff Works. http://www.howstuffworks.com/medical-marijuana.htm. Accessed on January 7, 2012.

This popular website provides a good overall introduction to the subject of medical marijuana.

"Info on Cannabis (Marijuana)." Centre for Addiction and Mental Health. http://www.camh.net/About_Addiction_Mental_Health/AMH101/top_searched_cannabis.html. Accessed on January 7, 2012.

This Canadian website is a rich source of information on all aspects of cannabis and its use as a recreational drug.

"Marijuana." MedlinePlus. http://www.nlm.nih.gov/medlineplus/marijuana.html. Accessed on December 4, 2011. This website, maintained by the U.S. National Library of Medicine, is a reliable source of information about every aspect of marijuana, including basic information, research, directories, organizations, and resources.

"Marijuana." National Institute on Drug Abuse. http://www.drugabuse.gov/tib/marijuana.html. Accessed on December 4, 2011. The National Institute on Drug Abuse issues fact sheets that are updated regularly on a variety of substance abuse issues. The fact sheets provide reliable information, primarily on medical aspects of the drug.

"Marijuana: Addiction and Other Issues." University of Wisconsin–Madison, University Health Services. http://www.uhs.wisc.edu/health-topics/alcohol-and-drugs/marijuana-addiction-and-other-issues.shtml. Accessed on January 7, 2012. This fact sheet provides a nice general review of the risk and character of addiction to and physical dependence on marijuana.

"Marijuana Use and Its Effects." WebMD. http://www.webmd.com/mental-health/marijuana-use-and-its-effects. Accessed on January 7, 2012. This website provides basic information on the physiological and psychological effects of marijuana, with some useful links to other sources on the subject.

"Medical Marijuana." DrugWarFacts.org. http://drugwarfacts.org/cms/?q=node/54. Accessed on January 7, 2012. This is an enormously valuable website because of the extensive list of references it provides for all aspects related to the therapeutic use of marijuana.

"Medical Marijuana." ProCon.org. http://medicalmarijuana. procon.org/view.resource.php?resourceID=000143. Accessed on December 3, 2011.

This timeline provides an excellent review of the history of medical marijuana, with relatively little information about other uses or issues related to the drug.

"Medical Marijuana Program." California Department of Public Health. http://www.cdph.ca.gov/programs/mmp/Pages/Medical %20Marijuana%20Program.aspx. Accessed on January 7, 2012.

This website provides a variety of information regarding the medical marijuana (MM) program in California, including related regulations and statutes, data and statistics, funding, patient advocacy groups, organizations, and information about the MM program in the state.

Nelson, Robert A. "A History of Hemp." rexresearch.com http://www.rexresearch.com/hhist/hhist1.htm. Accessed on December 12, 2011.

This website provides an excellent introduction to the history of hemp uses dating from the Neolithic period to the early Renaissance.

NORML. "About Marijuana." http://norml.org/marijuana. Accessed on December 8, 2011.

This website, hosted by perhaps the best known and most respected of all organizations striving to decriminalize the use of marijuana, provides extensive basic information about the personal, medical, and industrial use of cannabis, as well as information about drug testing and a list of endorsements for the organization's position on marijuana use.

Office of National Drug Control Policy. "What Americans Need to Know about Marijuana." https://www.ncjrs.gov/ ondcppubs/publications/pdf/mj_rev.pdf. Accessed on December 5, 2011.

This government publication claims that Americans are very much uninformed about the real threat that marijuana poses, and it explores five major myths about the drug and explains how existing federal policy can reduce the risk of harm to Americans caused by use of marijuana.

Rudgley, Richard. "Cannabis." The Encyclopedia of Psychoactive Substances. http://cannabis.net/hist/index.html. Accessed on January 7, 2012.

This long essay provides a complete overview of the role of cannabis products in human history.

Scheerer, Sebastian. "North American Bias and Non-American Roots of Cannabis Prohibition." http://www.bisdro.uni-bremen.de/boellinger/cannabis/04-schee.pdf. Accessed on December 6, 2011.

The author provides a brief review of efforts to criminalize the use of cannabis a number of years before such a movement began in the United States.

"Smoking and How to Quit." womenshealth.gov. http://womenshealth.gov/smoking-how-to-quit/other-forms-tobacco-nicotine-marijuana/marijuana.cfm. Accessed on December 4, 2011.

This website focuses on the effects of marijuana on women's health and provides extensive information and resources related to the drug and ways to stop using it.

Stafford, Ned. "Synthetic Cannabis Mimic Found In Herbal Incense." Cannabis Culture. http://www.cannabisculture.com/v2/news/synthetic-cannabis-mimic-found-in-herbal-incense. Accessed on December 16, 2011.

This website reports on the discovery of a synthetic drug developed at Clemson University in the mid-1990s with a potency at least four times that of THC in "incense products" being sold in Europe. The drug, known as JWH-018, has since been classified as a schedule I drug in the

United States, although it is still available legally in some parts of the world.

Szalavitz, Maia. "Is Marijuana Addictive? It Depends How You Define Addiction." http://healthland.time.com/2010/10/19/is-marijuana-addictive-it-depends-how-you-define-addiction/. Accessed on January 7, 2012.

This article takes a careful and detailed look at the question of marijuana addiction, with the major theme being that stated by the title of the article.

U.S. Drug Enforcement Administration. *The DEA Position on Marijuana.* http://www.justice.gov/dea/marijuana_position.pdf. Accessed on December 5, 2011.

This booklet outlines the position of the U.S. Drug Enforcement Administration on the use and legalization of marijuana both for general and for medical use. The booklet presents detailed descriptions and analyses of the status of marijuana law in a number of states.

West, David P. "Hemp and Marijuana: Myths and Realities." http://www.naihc.org/hemp_information/content/hemp.mj.html. Accessed on December 23, 2011.

This white paper was presented in 1998 on behalf of the North American Industrial Hemp Council to clarify the essential differences between hemp and marijuana as well as to argue for the importance of hemp as an industrial product in the modern world.

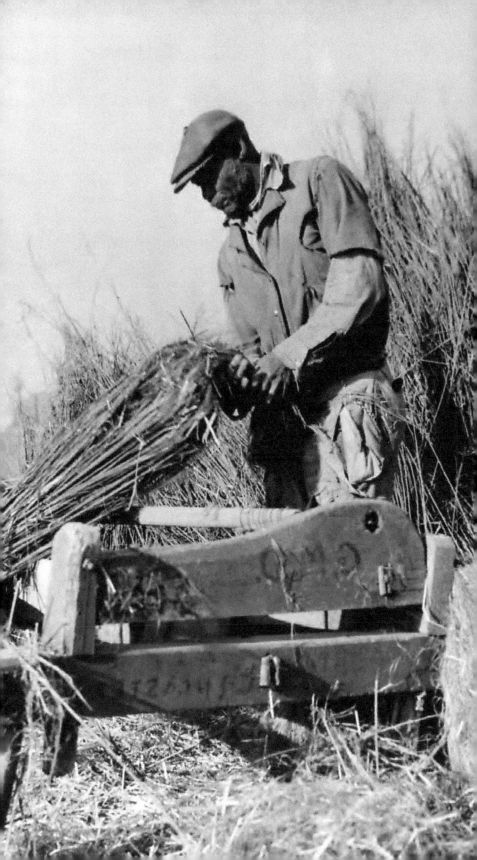

Introduction

Marijuana and the Cannabis plant from which it comes have been known to humans for thousands of years. During that time, the plant has had a variety of uses, for the production of fibers, in the form of hemp; for the manufacture of oil, from the plant's seeds; and as a recreational drug, produced from the dried leaves, seeds, and stems of the plant. The history of these three classes of products is long, complex, and often in dispute. The chronology provided here lists some of the most important of those dates, with points of dispute mentioned where they are appropriate.

ca. 6000 BCE   Reports of cannabis seeds being used for food.

ca. 4000 BCE   Reports of hemp being used for the production of textiles in China and Turkmenistan. Some authorities argue that hemp is the first plant material cultivated specifically for use in the production of textiles.

2737 BCE   Claims that cannabis products are used for medicinal purposes. The Chinese Emperor Shen Nung is reputed to have recommended the drug for treatment of beri-beri,

---

Hemp has been widely used by humans throughout history, and it was once a major cash crop in the United States. Currently, it is illegal to grow hemp in the United States. (Public Records Division, Kentucky Department for Libraries and Archives)

gout, constipation, "female weakness," malaria, and other medical conditions. Most evidence suggests that Shen Nung was a mythological character, and that what is reputed to be his most important work, *Shen-nung pen ts'ao ching (Divine Husbandman's Materia Medica)* dates instead to the fourth century BCE.

ca. 2000 BCE   Egyptian healers reputedly recommend marijuana for the treatment of sore eyes.

ca. 1700 BCE   Archaeological evidence suggests that smoked marijuana was used as an aid during childbirth in Judea, with the practice probably being widespread at the time throughout the Middle East.

ca. 1000 BCE   The first recorded use of the drink known as bhang, made from the leaves and flowers of the female cannabis plant, during Hindu religious ceremonies. The drink is still popular today for its mild intoxicant effects.

ca. 500 BCE   The first certain identification of hemp, in any form, is recorded near Stuttgart, Germany. The fiber begins to spread throughout Europe shortly thereafter and eventually becomes an essential textile material.

446 BCE   The Greek historian Herodotus writes of a Scythian ceremony in which participants throw hemp seed on a hot stone inside a tent and inhale the fumes produced, causing them such joy that "they would howl with pleasure."

ca. 200 BCE   First reported use of hemp for the production of paper during the Western Han dynasty in China. By this time in history, the plant was also being used widely for the manufacture of canvas sails, the name of which, "canvas," comes from the Latin word *cannabis*, the Greek word *kannabis*, and even earlier terms for "hemp."

70 CE   Pedacius Dioscorides, a physician in the army of the Roman emperor Nero, compiles a pharmacopeia that lists marijuana as a useful herb for the treatment of a variety of disorders, including earache.

ca. 100 CE   Chinese scholar and government official Ts'ai Lun manufactures paper out of "rags, fish nets, bark of trees, and hemp well prepared," earning him the title of "the inventor of paper."

Second century CE   The famous Roman physician, Galen, writes about cannabis in his *De Alimentorum Facultatibus* (*On the Properties of Foodstuffs*), pointing out that when toasted and eaten with drinks, they are hard to digest, but, upon absorption by the body, the drug "hits the head, if it is ingested in too much quantity in a short time, and sends hot, in the meantime pharmaceutical fumes to it."

ca. 400   Cannabis cultivated for the first time in England at Old Buckeham Mare in Norfolk County.

1151   The first paper mill using hemp as a raw material is built by Moorish officials at Xatvia, Spain. Papermaking using hemp spreads throughout Europe with the first mills opening in France in 1189, Italy in 1268, Germany in 1390, Holland in 1428, Switzerland in 1433, and England in 1494.

1533   King Henry VIII decrees that all landowners who farm more than 60 acres are required to include at least a quarter of an acre for the growing of hemp.

1545   Spaniards introduce cannabis growing to the world, establishing a hemp farm in Chile for the production of hemp for use in ropemaking. By 1564, King Philip of Spain decrees that hemp is to be grown in Spanish possessions throughout the New World.

1606   French apothecary Louis Hébert plants the first commercial crop of *Cannabis sativa* in Nova Scotia.

1619   The first law in the United States mandating that farmers plant hemp is adopted in Jamestown Colony, Virginia. The law is imposed because of the huge demand for hemp in Great Britain. Similar laws are soon passed in Connecticut (1637) and Massachusetts (1639).

1753   *Cannabis sativa* is first classified by the Swedish taxonomist Linnaeus.

1758   French biologist Jean-Baptiste de Lamarck classifies a second species of cannabis, *C. indica.* Most biologists now considered *C. indica* to be a subspecies of *C. sativa.*

1790s   Both George Washington and Thomas Jefferson promote the growth of hemp because of its many uses.

1839   Irish-born, Calcutta-based physician William Brooke O'Shaughnessy publishes the first scientific article on the medical uses of cannabis based on his experiences with use of the drug among native Indians.

1860   The Ohio State Medical Society establishes a committee to study the medical effects of *C. indica.* The committee reports on beneficial effects of the drug, including the cure of neuralgic pain, dysmenorrhea, uterine hemorrhage, hysteria, delirium tremens, mania, palsy, whooping cough, and infantile convulsions.

1870   For the first time, the U.S. Pharmacopeia lists cannabis as a medicine.

1895   The India Hemp Commission issues a report on the use of cannabis by native Indians and finds that it has some medical benefits and "no evil results at all."

1895   Probably the first use of the word *marihuana* for the cannabis plant, by supporters of Pancho Villa in Sonora, Mexico.

1906   U.S. Congress passes the Pure Food and Drug Act, the first major piece of legislation designed to provide some monitoring of foods and drugs sold in the United States. The minimum requirement established for many drugs, including marijuana, was that products containing such drugs be labeled to indicate the drug's presence.

1911   South Africa bans the use of cannabis, largely because its use by mine workers resulted in a reduction in their productivity.

1911   Massachusetts becomes the first state in the United States to ban the use of cannabis.

1912   The First International Opium Conference is held in the Hague, Netherlands, at which the first international drug control treaty (The International Opium Convention, or The Hague Convention) is adopted. A ban on cannabis is considered but not included in the final treaty.

1914   U.S. Congress passes the Harrison Narcotics Tax Act, which regulates and sets taxes on the production and use of opiates. No mention of marijuana is made in the act. (But see 1934.)

1915   The state of Utah passes an antimarijuana law, apparently based on the tendency of young Mormon missionaries returning from their time in Mexico to bring back the custom of marijuana smoking with them.

1915   California outlaws marijuana.

1916   The U.S. Department of Agriculture (USDA) issues Bulletin 404, which calls for greater cultivation of hemp, pointing out that each acre planted to hemp produces as much pulp as would be obtained from more than four acres of trees.

1919   Texas outlaws marijuana.

1923   South African delegates to the United Nations ask that cannabis be added to the list of dangerous drugs included in the Hague Convention. Support for this position comes from Italy, Egypt, and Turkey.

1924   The Second International Opium Conference in Geneva agrees to list cannabis as a narcotic under terms of the Hague Convention.

1928   The UK Dangerous Drugs Acts makes the use of marijuana illegal in the United Kingdom.

1931   Secretary of the Treasury Andrew Mellon appoints Harry J. Anslinger first commissioner of the new Federal Bureau of Narcotics. Over the next three decades, Anslinger becomes the foremost proponent for the criminalization of marijuana use.

1933   A report commissioned by the commanding general of the U.S. Panama Canal Department concludes that "[mariajuana] is not a 'habit forming' drug in the sense that the derivatives of opium and cocaine are such drugs, as there are no symptoms of deprivation following its withdrawal."

1934   Because marijuana was not mentioned in the Harrison Act of 1914, the National Conference of Commissioners on Uniform State Laws recommends a Uniform State Narcotic Drug Act, which they suggest that all states adopt so that there will be a common policy on marijuana prosecutions throughout the nation. At first, only nine states adopt the act, and it is soon superseded by the 1937 Marihuana Tax Act.

1936   An international conference in Geneva adopts the Convention for the Suppression of the Illicit Traffic in Dangerous Drugs (the Trafficking Convention). The United States declines to sign the treaty because it regards its conditions as too weak.

1936   The film *Tell Your Children*, describing the consequences of marijuana use, is released. The film eventually becomes famous under the title *Reefer Madness* and is re-created in a 2005 made-for-television film and a 2011 Broadway musical.

1937   U.S. Congress passes the Marihuana Tax Act, imposing a tax on anyone who "imports, manufactures, produces, compounds, sells, deals in, dispenses, prescribes, administers, or gives away marihuana." Among other effects, the act essentially ends the growing of hemp in the United States.

1941   Cannabis is delisted from the American Pharmacopeia.

1941   President Franklin D. Roosevelt signs an order allowing production of hemp for industrial uses during World War II. The ban on hemp production is restored at the end of the war in 1945.

1943   The U.S. government produces a film and begins a campaign called Hemp for Victory, urging farmers to increase their production of hemp for war uses.

1944   The La Guardia Report, named after the mayor of New York City, concludes, among other findings, that "[t]he practice of smoking marihuana does not lead to addiction in the medical sense of the word . . . [m]arihuana is not the determining factor in the commission of major crimes . . . and [t]he publicity concerning the catastrophic effects of marihuana smoking in New York City is unfounded."

1951   An issue of the UN *Bulletin of Narcotic Drugs* (3[1]: 22–45) endorses an estimate of 200 million users of cannabis products worldwide.

1951   U.S. Congress passes the Boggs Amendment to the Harrison Act of 1914 (dealing with cocaine and opiates), providing for severe mandatory sentencing for the possession, sale, or use of narcotic drugs, including marijuana.

1956   The Narcotics Control Act increases mandatory fines and sentences beyond those set by the Boggs Amendment of 1951.

1957   The tax consequences of growing hemp become so onerous that the last hemp farm in the United States, located in Wisconsin, ceases cultivation of the product.

1968   A U.K. report on marijuana use chaired by the Baroness Wootton concludes that marijuana use does no more harm than tobacco or alcohol use and recommends that all penalties for possession and use of small amounts of the drug be repealed.

1969   In Mill Valley, California, the first organization in the United States is formed to decriminalize marijuana. The organization, originally called Le Mar, is later renamed Amorphia.

1970   The Controlled Substances Act is an effort to revise and update the complicated series of laws that deal with illegal drugs. One of its main provisions is the creation of drug "schedules" that specify the potential for abuse and medical value of various drugs. Marijuana is listed as a schedule I drug, the highest and most dangerous category.

1970   Public interest attorney R. Keith Stroup founds the National Organization for the Reform of Marijuana Laws (NORML) in Washington, DC.

1971   The English government ignores the recommendations of the Wootton Committee (1968) and classifies marijuana as a class B drug, banning its use for all medical purposes.

1972   The National Commission on Marijuana and Drug Abuse (the Shafer Commission), created by Public Law 91-513 to study marijuana abuse in the United States, issues its final report entitled *Marijuana: A Signal of Misunderstanding*. The commission recommends the decriminalization of marijuana.

1972   Amorphia sponsors state Proposition 19 in California, calling for the decriminalization of small amounts of marijuana for personal use. The proposition fails with a vote of 35.5 percent "yes" to 66.5 percent "no."

1972   Oregon becomes the first state in the United States to decriminalize the use of marijuana.

1973   President Richard Nixon issues Reorganization Plan No. 2 of 1973, transferring most responsibility for the enforcement of federal drug laws from the Department of the Treasury to a new entity, the Drug Enforcement Administration (DEA) in the Department of Justice.

1974   Amorphia becomes the California chapter of NORML.

1976   President Gerald Ford bans all federal funding for research on the medical benefits of marijuana.

1976   The U.S. government establishes the Compassionate Investigational New Drug program that allows a select group of patients to use marijuana for medical purposes. President George W. Bush terminated the program for new participants in 1992 and, as of early 2012, four patients remained in the program, which is administered by the University of Mississippi.

1976   The Dutch government adopts a "policy of expediency" with regard to the use of marijuana, which, while not legalizing the drug, instructs police and prosecutors to ignore retail sale to adults as long as the circumstances of the sale do not constitute a public nuisance.

1977   In a message to the U.S. Congress on August 2, 1977, President Jimmy Carter endorses the findings of the Shafer Commission and famously says that "Penalties against possession of a drug should not be more damaging to an individual than the use of the drug itself."

1982   Newt Gingrich, later speaker of the House of Representatives, writes to the *Journal of the American Medical Association* (*JAMA*) to say that "patients have a right to obtain marijuana legally, under medical supervision, from a regulated source."

1983   The administration of President Ronald Reagan encourages all academic researchers to destroy all research on cannabis conducted between 1966 and 1976.

1988   U.S. Drug Enforcement Administration (DEA) law judge Francis Young finds that marijuana "in strict medical terms is far safer than many foods we consume" and, therefore, the drug should be transferred from schedule I to schedule II. (DEA administrative law judges are judges assigned to hold hearings on and rule on enforcement and regulatory cases brought by the DEA.)

1991   The U.S. Court of Appeals for the District of Columbia upholds Judge Young's decision on marijuana, but DEA administrator Robert C. Bonner exercises his right to reject the recommended decision "with a vengeance."

1996   Voters in Arizona and California approve initiatives allowing the use of marijuana for the treatment of medical conditions. Officials of the Clinton administration announce that the actions in Arizona and California are in conflict with federal law, and any person acting under the provisions of either act will be subject to federal prosecution.

1997   The Arizona legislature passes legislation prohibiting any physician from acting under the recently passed medical marijuana bill until the use of marijuana had been approved by federal legislation, essentially invalidating voters' actions in the 1996 election.

1997   An editorial in the prestigious *New England Journal of Medicine* calls the prohibition on the use of marijuana for treating certain medical conditions "misguided, heavy-handed, and inhumane."

1998   Voters in Alaska, Oregon, and Washington approve ballot measures removing state penalties for the use of marijuana for medical purposes.

1999   The U.S. Institute of Medicine issues its report called *Marijuana and Medicine: Assessing the Science Base* on the medical uses of marijuana.

2001   Portugal decriminalizes the use of marijuana for personal use.

2001   Canada became the world's first country to regulate the use of marijuana, as legislation that allows people with serious illnesses to possess marijuana comes into force.

2004   The citizens of Montana vote about 2:1 to allow the use of marijuana for medical purposes. In 2011, both houses of the state legislature vote to repeal that vote, essentially eliminating the use of medical marijuana in the state.

2005   In the case of *Gonzales v. Raich*, the U.S. Supreme Court rules that Congress may criminalize the production and use of home-grown marijuana, even in states where the use of the drug for medical purposes is legal.

2006   The U.S. Food and Drug Administration (FDA) issues a policy statement saying that there are "no sound scientific studies" that marijuana has any medical benefits and that, in fact, the drug has "high potential for abuse."

2009   Mexico decriminalizes the use of marijuana for personal use.

2010   The Czech cabinet approves decriminalization of drug possession for personal use.

2011   Representative Barney Frank (D-MA) introduces legislation (H.R. 2306) that would remove marijuana from the list of controlled substances (i.e., decriminalize marijuana in the United States).

2011   Representative Frank also introduces legislation (H.R. 1983) requiring the Secretary of Health and Human Services to recommend a relisting of marijuana under some category other than schedule I or II and declares that federal regulations shall not be construed to conflict with the decisions of individual states to permit the medical use of marijuana.

2011   In response to a petition filed in 2002 requesting that marijuana be rescheduled as a drug of less than schedule I, Michele M. Leonhart, administrator of the Drug Enforcement Administration, denies the request, indicating that marijuana has "a high potential for abuse. . . . no currently accepted medical use in treatment in the United States. . . . [and] accepted safety for use under medical supervision."

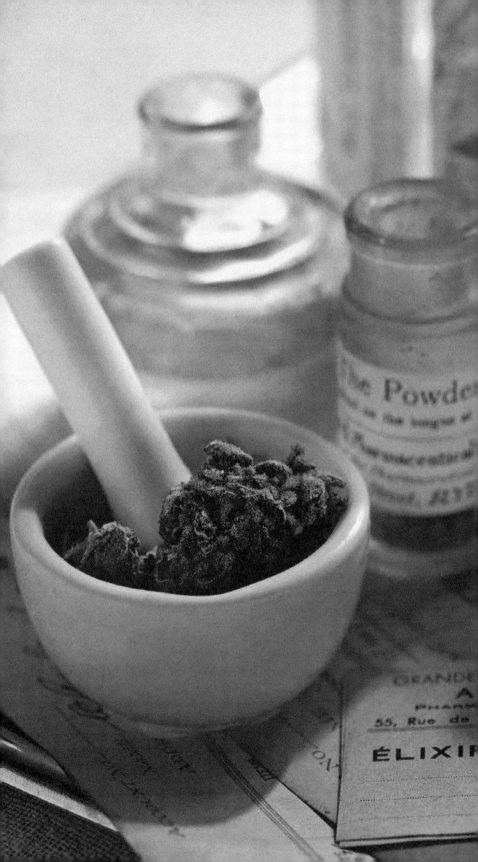

Glossary

Introduction

Discussions of marijuana may involve terminology that is unfamiliar to the average person. In some cases, the terms used are scientific, technical, or medical expressions used most commonly by professionals in the field. In other cases, the terms may be part of the "street slang" that users themselves employ in talking about the drugs they consume, the paraphernalia associated with drugs, or the experiences that accompany marijuana use. This glossary lists and defines a few of the terms needed to understand explanations provided in this book.

accepted medical use A term used in the Controlled Substances Act of 1970 not defined in the act, but later defined by the Drug Enforcement Agency to mean any drug (1) whose chemistry is known and is reproducible, (2) has had adequate safety studies, (3) for which there are adequate and well-controlled studies proving efficacy, (4) has been accepted by qualified experts, and (5) for which scientific evidence is widely available.

blind trial A research study in which a patient does not know whether he or she is receiving the experimental treatment or a placebo. *Also see* **double blind trial.**

A few of the many products that can be made from hemp include yarn, string, webbing, lip balm, hand oil, moisturizing wash, foot rub, pet products, cereals, nuts, fruit bars, and other food products. (Lew Robertson/Fuse)

cannabinoid   Any one of a group of compounds that include cannabinol and the active constituents of cannabis.

cannabinol   A psychoactive substance found in plants in the genera *Cannabis*. Its systematic name is 6,6,9-trimethyl-3-pentyl-benzo[c]chromen-1-ol, and its chemical formula, $C_{21}H_{26}O_2$.

clinical trial   A research study conducted to determine the effect of some new experimental treatment, such as a new drug or a new vaccine.

controlled substance   Any substance listed under schedule I through V of the Controlled Substances Act of 1970, or a precursor of one of those substances.

decriminalization   Removal or reduction of penalties associated with some previously illegal act, such as reductions in penalties for possession or use of marijuana.

double blind trial   A research study in which neither patients nor researchers know whether subjects of the study are receiving the experimental treatment or a placebo.

dronabinol   A synthetic cannabinoid used for anorexia with patients suffering from HIV/AIDS as well as nausea and vomiting associated with chemotherapy. Trade name: Marinol.

drug diversion   Providing a drug to an individual who is not authorized to use it.

efficacy   The degree to which a substance produces some effect expected of it.

gateway theory   The hypothesis that the use of one drug increases one's tendency to experiment with other drugs.

hashish   A product made from compressed trichomes (resin glands) of the cannabis plant, usually made available in the form of a sticky, often thick, paste that can be burned, smoked, or cooked in foods, with considerably more potent psychoactive effects than marijuana.

hemp   A tough, coarse fiber made from the cannabis plant; used to make textiles, canvas, paper, rope, and other items.

marijuana A greenish, brown, or gray mixture of the shredded leaves, flowers, and stems of the cannabis plant, smoked as a cigarette or in a special kind of pipe.

medical necessity A legal doctrine that one may be permitted to carry out a medical act that is otherwise illegal if, in so doing, a greater harm is prevented.

narcotic A drug that in moderate doses relieves pain and dulls the senses, but in greater doses may cause stupor, coma, convulsions, and/or death.

nostrum A type of medication whose composition is secret and for which scientific evidence of its efficacy does not exist.

peer-reviewed study A research study whose methodology and results have been examined by other experts in the same field to decide if the study is worthy of being published.

potency The strength of a drug; in the case of marijuana, an indirect measure of the amount of tetrahydrocannabinol (THC) in a sample of the drug.

psychoactive Capable of producing mind-altering affects, such as changes in mood or perception.

psychotropic *See* **psychoactive**.

purity The amount of a desired component, such as pure cannabis, present in a mixture that also contains impurities.

sinsemilla From the Spanish *sin* ("without") *semilla* ("seed"); a form of marijuana that has a high percentage of THC and is, hence, much more potent than marijuana made of a mixture of plant parts.

slippery slope The argument that once an individual or society has taken the first step in some undesirable action (such as permitting the use of marijuana), it then becomes much more likely that worse eventualities will follow (such as permitting the use of other, more dangerous drugs).

Spice   The common name used for synthetic cannabis; also known as Fire 'n' Ice, Genie, K2, PEP Spice, Solar Flare, Spice Diamond, Spice Gold, and Yucatan Fire.

street slang   Some of the terms in the everyday vernacular used to describe marijuana, including Afghan, bhang, Buddha grass, dope, draw, gage, ganja, gangster, grass, herb, Jane, jive, joint, kiff, loco weed, Mary, Mary Jane, MJ, Mexican green, Panama red, pot, puff, reefer, roach, smoke, spliff, tea, Texas tea.

synthetic cannabis   A combination of natural herbs and synthetic chemicals that, when ingested, produce psychoactive effects similar to those of natural cannabis.

tetrahydrocannabinol   *See* **THC.**

THC   An abbreviation for tetrahydrocannabinol, the chemical compound responsible for the psychoactive effects produced by the ingestion of cannabis. The compound is commonly known as delta-9-tetrahydrocannabinol (Δ9-THC).

trichome   A fine hairy-like projection from the epidermal cells of a plant which, in the cannabis plant, contain the chemical substance, THC, responsible for the psychoactive effects of the drug.

Index

About the Author

David E. Newton holds an associate's degree in science from Grand Rapids (Michigan) Junior College, a B.A. in chemistry (with high distinction), an M.A. in education from the University of Michigan, and an Ed.D. in science education from Harvard University. He is the author of more than 400 textbooks, encyclopedias, resource books, research manuals, laboratory manuals, trade books, and other educational materials. He taught mathematics, chemistry, and physical science in Grand Rapids, Michigan, for 13 years; was professor of chemistry and physics at Salem State College in Massachusetts for 15 years; and was adjunct professor in the College of Professional Studies at the University of San Francisco for 10 years. Previous books for ABC-CLIO include *Global Warming* (1993), *Gay and Lesbian Rights: A Resource Handbook* (1994, 2009), *The Ozone Dilemma* (1995), *Violence and the Mass Media* (1996), *Environmental Justice* (1996, 2009), *Encyclopedia of Cryptology* (1997), *Social Issues in Science and Technology: An Encyclopedia* (1999), *DNA Technology* (2009), and *Sexual Health* (2010). Other recent books include *Physics: Oryx Frontiers of Science Series* (2000), *Sick!* (4 volumes; 2000), *Science, Technology, and Society: The Impact of Science in the 19th Century* (2 volumes; 2001), *Encyclopedia of Fire* (2002), *Molecular Nanotechnology: Oryx Frontiers of Science Series* (2002), *Encyclopedia of Water* (2003), *Encyclopedia of Air* (2004), *The New Chemistry* (6 volumes; 2007), *Nuclear Power* (2005), *Stem Cell Research* (2006), *Latinos in the Sciences, Math, and Professions* (2007), and *DNA*

Evidence and Forensic Science (2008). He has also been an updating and consulting editor on books and reference works, including *Chemical Compounds* (2005), *Chemical Elements* (2006), *Encyclopedia of Endangered Species* (2006), *World of Mathematics* (2006), *World of Chemistry* (2006), *World of Health* (2006), *UXL Encyclopedia of Science* (2007), *Alternative Medicine* (2008), *Grzimek's Animal Life Encyclopedia* (2009), *Community Health* (2009), and *Genetic Medicine* (2009).